C000270643

Your Healthy House

Every patient is unique, as is every illness. This book is intended as a source of information only. Readers are urged to work in partnership with a qualified, experienced practitioner before undertaking (or refraining from) any treatments listed in these pages.

© Copyright 2003. What Doctors Don't Tell You Limited

First published in various editions of **PROOF!** and **WDDTY**. Editor and co-publisher: Lynne McTaggart. Publisher: Bryan Hubbard

No part of this publication may be reproduced or transmitted in any form or by any means, electronic or mechanical, including recording, photocopy, computerised or electronic storage or retrieval system, without permission granted in writing from the publisher.

While every care is taken in preparing this material, the publisher cannot accept any responsibility for any damage or harm caused by any treatment, advice or information contained in this publication. You should consult a qualified practitioner before undertaking any treatment.

ISBN: 0-9534734-7-3

A What Doctors Don't Tell You Publication

YOUR HEALTHY HOUSE

Edited by Lynne McTaggart

To all our readers—
and their good health

Contents

Preface

We all take comfort from the ancient adage that our home is our castle, a safe refuge from the insults of the world. And while, indeed, it may be a haven for the family, it is sadly far from being a safe one.

Pollutants from gases and pesticides, electromagnetic fields (EMFs) from electrical gadgets and power lines, and subtle environmental changes from seemingly benign household items are all byproducts of the age of convenience and comfort.

Our constant exposure to these pollutants and chemicals can cause a spectrum of illnesses that affect us and the rest of our family, ranging from cancers to those hard-to-define feelings of depression or lack of energy.

So, our haven from a hostile world may, in fact, hold the key to our own state of wellbeing.

Your Healthy House is a compilation of all that **What Doctors Don't Tell You** and **PROOF!** have researched and published over the past 12 years. The coverage is broad, and encompasses every type and source of pollutant, EMF, pesticide and the like that you are likely to encounter in your day-to-day life.

Not only does this collection include the unsuspected pollutants in your home, it also gives you the chapter and verse on the chemicals in the toiletries we use, including toothpaste and cosmetics, and those in found in household cleaners.

The radiation risks of microwave ovens and mobile phones are also described, with all the supporting scientific evidence and references.

All of this may seem like depressing reading. What, you may ask yourself, can one individual do about health hazards that are not being controlled by the various regulatory bodies?

The good news is that, if those bodies with the remit to ensure our safety cannot, or will not, perform their duties, you as an individual can still do much to reduce your own exposure to these risks. *Your Healthy House* not only tells you all about the dangers, but it also suggests alternatives you can use, and steps you can take, to counter these hazards.

While we cannot guarantee that everyone will be completely safe from these dangers of modern living, we know that your risk will be reduced to much safer levels if you are able to follow most of the recommendations in this book.

Your home might then be deserving of your trust that it is a safe haven from a polluted world.

There are many people we need to thank in preparing this book. Invaluable contributions have been made by Pat Thomas, Tony Edwards, Tony Lees, Joseph Hattersley and Simon Best, while Clive Couldwell has compiled and edited the articles.

To all of them we give our thanks because, without them, we could not produce **What Doctors Don't Tell You** and **PROOF!** and, without you, our readers, there would be no point to researching this material in the first place.

So thank you for buying this book, and we truly hope it serves you well.

Lynne McTaggart

Chapter 1
The dangers inside your home

We spend an estimated 90 per cent of our lives indoors and, much of that time, inside our own homes. Once we've shut our front door, we tend to see our living space as a refuge, imagining it to be a safe haven from the world outside—and certainly less polluted.

But surprisingly, it's not—in fact, quite the reverse. A recent report by the normally conservative US Environmental Protection Agency (EPA) stated: "Indoor air pollution in residences, offices, schools and other buildings is . . . one of the most serious potential environmental risks to health."

Ever since the oil crisis of 1973, when "save energy" became the new mantra, houses have been made increasingly airtight. At the same time, many new materials have found their way into our homes, developed by the building and home-furnishing industries. These new substances are all synthetic and many are potentially toxic, causing one industry expert to describe our indoor air quality as a "chemical soup".

"Consumers are largely ignorant of the health threat posed by these new materials, relatively few of which have been tested for toxicity," says environmental architect Paula Baker. "But there is growing concern that chronic, low-level toxic exposure is on the increase, resulting in symptoms that are often falsely attributed to the normal ageing process" (Baker P et al., Prescriptions for a Healthy House, Santa Fe, NM: Inword Press, 1998).

One long-term study found that indoor air often contains more hazardous chemicals than outdoor air—even in highly industrialised areas. Between 1979 and 1995, the EPA compared indoor and outdoor pollution in three different locations: industrialised Bayonne, New

Jersey; semi-industrialised Greensboro, North Carolina; and rural Devil's Lake, North Dakota. By means of an automatic pump attached to their chests, the air of some 355 people was sampled as they went about their daily activities.

In a typical day at work and at home, these people were found to breathe at least two to five times more hazardous chemicals when indoors than if they had sat in their gardens. This was true even if the people lived within a mile of a source of industrial air pollution, as in New Jersey. In North Carolina and North Dakota, the results were even more striking: indoor air chemicals were between five and 10 times higher than the levels outside (Environ Res, 1987; 43: 290–307).

In Britain, related studies by Dr Geoffrey Llewellyn and colleagues at the Building Research Establishment (BRE) came to similar conclusions, finding that in semi-rural Avon, air quality was, on average, 10 times worse indoors than outdoors. His team found over 200 indoor chemicals, of which 80 were judged to have significant adverse health consequences (*BRE Report no 299*, Construction Research Corporation Ltd, 1996).

As a result, the BRE now recommends that houses should have a complete air change every two hours. In today's well-sealed, energy-efficient dwellings, air changes average less than half that. Chronic exposure to toxins in the indoor environment has now been linked to a vast spectrum of illnesses, ranging from asthma, chronic sinus infections, headaches, insomnia, anxiety, fatigue and joint pain to full-blown multiple chemical sensitivities (Publ Health Rep, 1998; 113: 398–409). The authors of this particular study, two doctors from the prestigious Massachusetts General Hospital in Boston, lay the blame on "the explosion in the use of chemicals in building construction and furnishing materials over the past four decades".

Indoor air pollutants can be classified into five main categories: volatile organic compounds (VOCs); toxic byproducts of combustion; pesticides; electromagnetic field pollution; and naturally occurring substances.

Volatile organic compounds (VOCs)

The biggest group is volatile organic compounds. Derived from petrochemicals, VOCs readily release vapours at room temperature in a process called "outgassing". VOCs are found in a multitude of materials used in the building and furnishing of today's average home—plywood, particle board, wood panelling, insulation, adhesives, carpets, paints, finishes and synthetic fabrics. Even many of the modern cleaning materials we use contain VOCs.

The distinctive smell of a new house is primarily caused by VOCs outgassing from the building materials, paints and furnishings. As with other pollutants, the extent and nature of the effects on your health depend on many factors, including the level of exposure and length of time exposed. Eye and respiratory tract irritation, headaches, dizziness, visual disorders and memory impairment are among the immediate symptoms that some people have experienced soon after exposure to VOCs.

Benzene and formaldehyde are the two major toxic VOCs. Indoor formaldehyde is gradually being recognised as a severe health hazard, even by such august bodies as the American Lung Association, which now recommends that formaldehyde levels should not exceed 0.1 parts per million. However, it is estimated that about half the US population is exposed to concentrations above this figure (Thrasher J, Broughton A, *The Poisoning of Our Homes and Workplaces*, Seadora, 1989).

In Europe, the situation may not be much better. A recent study of Austrian homes found indoor air concentrations of formaldehyde above the US threshold and, in some houses, 10 times higher (Cent Eur J Publ Health, 1997; 5: 127–30).

Formaldehyde is a colourless gas emitted by many construction materials and related products such as glues, resins and preservatives. In the fabric of buildings, the most significant sources of formaldehyde are likely to be in plywood and the adhesives used to bond pressed-wood building materials.

Urea-formaldehyde resins are found in wood products that are intended for indoor use which, paradoxically, emit more formaldehyde gas than the phenol-formaldehyde resins contained in products intended for exterior use. Certain foam-insulating materials, once widely used in housing construction, also contain large amounts of formaldehyde. They were banned in the US in 1985, and so, with the passage of time, they are unlikely to still be outgassing.

Although formaldehyde has been shown to cause cancer in animals, there is no definitive evidence linking it to cancer in humans. Other health hazards attributed to formaldehyde include skin rashes, watery eyes, breathing difficulties and burning sensations in the eyes, throat and nasal passages. It can also trigger asthma attacks.

Most people will react to formaldehyde when the levels are in the range of 0.1–1.1 parts per million. If the initial exposure is relatively high, some people may acquire a reduced tolerance to formaldehyde so that even low-level exposure at a later date will cause reactions.

People who develop permanent health problems as a result of formaldehyde exposure often relate the onset of their symptoms to a flu-like illness, which is usually misdiagnosed as a viral infection. Because formaldehyde is an immune-system sensitiser, it may cause multiple allergies and sensitivities to entirely unrelated substances if exposure is chronic .

Benzene is a known human carcinogen, a major source of which is paint. Oil-based paints are generally considered to be more hazardous than water-based paints, although both contain VOCs. Some manufacturers have now responded to public concern by developing very-low-VOC paints—at prices comparable to the conventional variety.

A recent meta-analysis of mortality rates among painters and decorators in Britain showed significantly more deaths from cancer compared with the rest of the population. This was largely attributed to benzene in paint (Cancer Detect Prev, 1998; 22: 533–9).

Cigarettes contain benzene but, in the non-smoking home, benzene is primarily found not only in paint, but also in carpets. In fact, carpets are one of the major sources of both formaldehyde and benzene as well as many other chemicals. A typical carpet may contain more than 120 chemicals in its fibre-bonding material, dyes, backing glues, fire retardant, latex binder, fungicide and antistatic and stain-resisting treatments.

Outgassing is at its peak when the carpet is new, but it can persist for up to three years after installation. In the US, the carpet industry has been put on the defensive after a rash of complaints from consumers regarding respiratory and neurological reactions to new carpets. Ironically, in 1987, some of the most adverse reactions occurred in the very heart of the top US regulatory body, the EPA, when over a thousand employees complained of symptoms after new carpeting was installed in their Washington headquarters. Although the agency publicly denied any link between these health symptoms and the new flooring, over 25,000 square yards of carpet was removed.

In 1992, in response to public concern, the US carpet industry began the Green Tag programme—a PR initiative to reduce VOCs in its products. However, recent animal experiments by an independent laboratory has shown that supposedly low VOC carpets can still be highly toxic (Anderson Laboratories Report, August 1992).

Lead in housepaint

Chipped paint in old houses, particularly in Europe, can be an overlooked culprit of high lead levels in blood. The Environmental Defense Fund, based in Washington, has released a report which highlights the continuing dangers of lead in household paint.

Despite a 1921 treaty that banned interior paints with more than 2 per cent of lead carbonate or lead sulphate, old housing stock is still decorated with the paint, especially in Europe, the report states. Lead chromate remains largely unregulated, and exterior paint with lead is still sold in most countries outside of the US.

The report *Global Dimensions of Lead Poisoning* also points out the increasing levels of lead in the atmosphere. During the Industrial Revolution, annual production of lead was 100,000 tonnes, but this has risen to 5.5 million tonnes today. Developed nations account for 65 per cent of world consumption; the countries of Latin America, Eastern Europe and Africa have increased their consumption steadily. African consumption has risen by 300 per cent in the last 20 years.

Combustion gases

A second cause of pollution in the home arises from the byproducts of combustion. Open fires, ranges and stoves, space heaters and central heating boilers and furnaces are all sources of potentially toxic gases, such as nitrogen oxide or dioxide, hydrogen cyanide and carbon monoxide.

In a study of 47,000 chemically sensitive patients, it was found that the most adverse reactions were caused by gas stoves, hot-water heaters, and furnaces and boilers (Rae W, *Chemical Sensitivity*, vol 2, Lewis Publishers, 1994: 706). However, even a tiny, unvented gas pilot light produces a significant amount of fumes, mainly nitrogen dioxide. Such gases have recently been shown to cause problems even in non-chemically sensitive children (Int J Epidemiol, 1997; 26: 788–96), resulting in "significant increases in sore throat, colds and absences from school". As one might expect, children with asthma react more adversely (Am J Respir Crit Care Med, 1998; 158: 891–5).

Carbon monoxide is a colourless, odourless gas which, as is well known, will cause death at fairly modest levels. Less well known, however, is how toxic carbon monoxide can be at much lower doses, where it can have serious effects on higher cognitive functions such as memory, concentration and reasoning, according to a study at Israel's Hadassah University (Arch Neurol, 1998; 55: 845–8).

Chronic exposure to carbon monoxide can also result in multiple chemical sensitivities, as it interferes with the detoxification pathways in the liver, causing toxic overload. In the recent book *Why Your House May Endanger Your Health,* author Dr Alfred Zamm describes how gas kitchen ranges have been the hidden culprit in many cases of what he calls "housewife's malaise". Zamm says that a gas oven operating at 350 degrees F for one hour, because of the inevitable incomplete combustion, can cause levels of carbon monoxide and nitrogen dioxide three times higher than typically found in a Los Angeles smog.

This is consistent with the recent findings of two doctors at Boston's Brigham Young Hospital, who discovered links between the use of domestic gas appliances and the incidence of lung disease (Thorax, 1997; 52 [Suppl 3]: S58–62).

Pesticides

Insecticides and fungicides number among the major health hazards in the home. These are found mainly in carpets, paints and wood. Many such pesticides were developed as offshoots of military nerve gases. We tend to assume that, because they are licensed for use in the home, they have been rendered safe for humans and domestic animals. However, a recent US government report admitted that less than 10 per cent of the hundreds of pesticides in common use have been adequately tested for safety.

A recent study showed that combining pesticides can add considerably to their toxicity, making them up to 1600 times more potent (Science, 1996; 272: 1489–92). Pyrethroids become extremely toxic to humans as well as insects when combined with the petroleum-derived piperonyl butoxide, and can even cause severe liver damage.

In older houses, insecticides are often sprayed in roof spaces to control woodworm, and householders are now cautioned about venturing too soon into the area after spraying. But there are also significant amounts of pesticides in the living areas—particularly in carpets. Not only are carpets sprayed to keep away moths, but they also tend to collect residues of pesticides that are tracked in from the outdoors. In fact, an EPA study in Florida found some of the highest household pesticide residues in carpet dust (Environ Sci Technol, year?; 30: 3313–20).

Because of their proximity to the floor, this makes infants and young children particularly vulnerable, with potentially serious long-term consequences. In one study, children who had been exposed to insecticides had a greater risk of developing brain tumours and other cancers (Am J Epidemiol, 1979; 109: 309–19).

Electromagnetic fields

Only recently have electromagnetic fields (EMFs) in the home become a cause for concern. Studies have concentrated on the adverse effects of high-tension power lines, where the evidence, although hotly debated, has tended to demonstrate a carcinogenic effect.

In animal studies, frequencies between 15 and 60 Hz have been shown to alter cellular protein synthesis, disrupt RNA synthesis and reduce immune response (Adey RW, in Norden B, Ramel C, eds, *Interaction Mechanisms of Low-level Electromagnetic Fields in Living Systems*, Oxford: Oxford University Press, 1992). As a precaution, Paula Baker recommends that magnetic fields be kept to a minimum in the area we spend most of our time—around our beds.

Leukaemia scare

In the first such case in Europe, a Lancashire couple are suing the local power company for the death of their 13-year-old son of leukaemia. Furthermore, a group of residents in north London recently won a judicial review over the laying of a 275,000-volt cable under their streets.

Considerable evidence now shows that living near relatively low levels of magnetic fields from mains electricity or power lines can raise the chances of your child getting leukaemia by three or four times. In

1979, two American researchers, Nancy Wertheimer and Ed Leeper, published the first major Western study linking EMFs from power lines and domestic wiring configurations to an increase in childhood cancer (Am J Epidemiol, 1979; 109: 273–84).

Since then, the evidence has become stronger; today, the National Grid can no longer dismiss it and is being forced to defend itself against a barrage of enquiries from the public and the press, including threats of legal action.

There are now some 12 studies of residential exposure to EMFs, of which nine show an elevated risk of childhood cancer; the three studies which do not show such a risk have been criticised for the way they were put together.

Teslas are a measure of the density of magnetic fields. An average household level is 70 nanoteslas (nT = one-thousandth of a millionth Tesla); the level beneath power lines can rise to over 1000 nT. On average, the positive studies have found a significantly increased risk at 200–300 nT whereas the National Radiological Protection Board (NRPB) will only begin to investigate at a level of 1600 microtesla (μT = one-millionth of a Tesla), a difference of 5400–8000 times.

In the US, the situation is very different. Many researchers advocate a general policy of "prudent avoidance", recommending a number of safety measures to avoid excessive exposure. At least 10 states have requirements on the level of EMFs allowed in houses built near power lines. There is also considerable litigation over health-hazard claims from residential and occupational exposure.

Electrical and magnetic fields surround all electrical conductors, including power lines, appliances and the wiring in your house. EMFs comprise both electrical fields and magnetic fields. Electrical fields are determined by voltage, from 240 volts in houses to as much as 400,000 volts on main power lines, and are generally highest around high-voltage transmission lines. The fields are similar to the static electricity shock from a new carpet. Unless you live near a power line, this isn't a major problem since they can be shielded by trees and walls.

Magnetic fields are generated by electrical currents whenever you use electricity. These are more worrisome because they can travel through walls and can't be shielded against except by lead shielding, and carefully designed wiring and electrical equipment.

The crux of the argument over what levels of EMFs constitute a hazard concerns the difference between thermal and non-thermal effects, and the perception of their harm. All electrical fields generate the same type of energy as ordinary sunlight. Thermal effects refer to those that occur when tissue is heated to a specific level by a given frequency at a given intensity at which damage takes place. This is how a microwave cooks food.

Non-thermal effects are those that occur below and, in many cases, well below the level at which tissue-heating occurs. Many scientific papers have shown that non-thermal effects exist, a conclusion which is accepted by the NRPB and other orthodox scientists. Disagreement is over the level at which such effects actually become harmful.

Here, independent researchers and other concerned parties are at loggerheads with the NRPB, which does not yet accept the implications of the majority of residential results pointing to the at-risk onset level of 200–300 nT for childhood cancer. The NRPB is the UK's appointed body charged with advising the government and other official bodies, including the National Grid and the Health & Safety Executive. Yet, it continues to base any exposure guidance on levels relating to thermal levels or known levels of damage.

In September 1992, Drs Maria Feychting and Anders Ahlbom, at the Institute of Environmental Medicine at the Karolinska Institute in Stockholm, announced the results of a large-scale epidemiological study, which found that children exposed to average domestic EMFs of 300 nT or more had almost four times the rate of leukaemia than expected. The study has now been published in the American Journal of Epidemiology (1993; 138: 467–81).

The subjects were the approximately 500,000 people who had lived within 300 metres of the country's network of 220 and 400 kV power lines between 1960 and 1985, of whom 142 children developed cancer.

Probably one of the soundest studies to date in terms of methodology, the Swedish study established for the first time a clear dose–response correlation between level of magnetic field exposure and increased incidence of leukaemia. Children exposed to above 100 nT EMFs had two times, those exposed to above 200 nT nearly three times, and those exposed to over 300 nT nearly four times the incidence of leukaemia compared with those exposed to less than 100 nT. Similar results were obtained when exposure was defined by proximity to power lines.

Such was the impact of this and another study published at the same time, which also found a strong link with brain tumours in men occupationally exposed to EMFs (Cancer Causes Control, 1993; 4: 465–76), that the Swedish National Board for Industrial and Technical Development (NUTEK) formally announced that henceforth it "would act on the assumption that there is a connection between exposure to power frequency magnetic fields and cancer, in particular childhood cancer."

In addition, NUTEK has advocated a moratorium on erecting power lines creating fields of 200 nT near houses and school buildings until further guidance, currently being drafted.

Indeed, even Professor Richard Doll, who now chairs the NRPB's Advisory Group on Non-Ionising Radiation, has admitted that the Swedish study is significantly better controlled and designed than previous ones and, thus, has increased the pressure on his organisation to carry out equally well-controlled studies of its own.

This is now about to be attempted in the form of a five-year, £5 million study by the UK Coordinating Committee for Cancer Research (UKCCCR), chaired by Professor Doll and funded by several medical charities as well as the electrical and nuclear industries. However, although EMFs are one of the factors researchers will be considering, there is concern by some independent researchers that certain specific factors may not be measured.

Roger Coghill, who runs one of the UK's few independent consultancies on EMFs in Pontypool, Wales, has argued that, whereas the magnetic field has been the main parameter considered in exposure studies to date, electric fields may, in fact, be the more significant factor. At present, this measure is not incorporated into the UKCCCR study's protocol.

The Feychting and Ahlbom study corroborates previous research by the American Dr John Peters, who found a significant link between wiring configurations in the home and childhood leukaemia (Am J Epidemiol, 1991; 134: 923–7), and Dr David Savitz, who also observed a two- to threefold increased risk in homes where the estimated magnetics exceeded 250–300 nT (Am J Epidemiol, 1988; 128: 21–38).

This cut-off level of increased risk has generally been supported by other positive studies. Pooling the results of three Nordic studies, including the recent Swedish one, Ahlbom and Feychting show a consistent doubling of childhood leukaemia risk (Lancet, 20 Nov 1993). Nevertheless, the earlier studies, including Savitz's, have confused researchers because they showed a positive association between the power load of the overhead lines and distance from the home, but not with the measurements inside the homes of children who developed leukaemia (JAMA, 5 Aug 1992). This was the main reason that researchers rejected the earlier data.

Gerald Draper, director of the Childhood Cancer Research Group, spoke for the orthodox view when he argued that the "lack of consistency" among published studies and the absence of an "accepted biological explanation for such a relation" means that no causal relationship has been established, even though, given the results of the Swedish study, it could no longer be dismissed (BMJ, 9 Oct 1993).

A further dimension to the whole power lines/EMF concern is that childhood leukaemia is but one of the possible health hazards identified, albeit the most researched. Other studies have found links with depression, heart attack and suicide, as well as minor problems such as headaches, insomnia and irritability.

Dr Leonard Sagan, from the Electric Power Research Institute in Palo Alto, California, believes that the most important research on EMFs must attempt to isolate which kind of exposure causes damage. "We must understand . . . whether there is a threshold level of exposure (dose) that must be surpassed to produce effects, or whether there are 'windows of exposure' of intensity or frequency, within which EMF may cause an effect," he says.

Household power and cancer

A leaked report reveals that electrical household gadgets such as vacuum cleaners, ovens and food mixers can cause cancer. The report, prepared for the US government's radiation advisors, recommends safety limits for exposure to electromagnetic fields.

The National Council on Radiation Protection says that EMF exposure should never be higher than 0.2 μT. If introduced, this would mean that most household gadgets would be considered unsafe; vacuum cleaners and drills, for example, have a range of between 2 and 20 μT, food mixers between 0.6 and 10 μT, hairdryers between 0.01 and 7 μT, dishwashers between 0.6 and 3 μT, washing machines between 0.15 and 3 μT, and electric ovens between 0.15 and 0.5 μT.

Without these appliances on, general household levels of EMFs are considered safe, unless the home is within 25 metres or less of a power line. If it is, a 400 kV line 25 metres from the home will increase general EMF levels to 8 μT.

The report, prepared by an 11-man committee over nine years, points to research which shows that exposure to even weak EMFs can affect the production of the hormone melatonin; this, in turn, interferes with the formation of oestrogen receptors in the breast, which may be linked to breast cancer.

These startling conclusions may soon gather support. The American Environmental Protection Agency is working on its own report and says its findings will be similar. Swedish authorities are already proposing that new schools for children should not have exposure levels of more than 0.2 μT (New Sci, 7 Oct 1995).

Biological pollutants

Another category of major household pollutants is the naturally occurring insect and microbial life that chooses to share our homes with us—principally house-dust mites and moulds.

Mites are a major culprit in causing allergies. They feed on skin cells and breed in mattresses, pillows, carpets and upholstery. There are an estimated 100,000 of them in every square yard of carpet.

However, while dust mites have long been cited as the cause of childhood allergies, new research evidence suggests that early exposure to bacteria in house dust is protective, not damaging.

The results of the study throw into question all the conventional wisdom of how to 'protect' babies and, indeed, suggest that the aggressive hygiene measures of modern societies may be partly responsible for the increase in atopic diseases.

Investigators analysed the house dust from the homes of 61 babies aged 9–24 months, who had had at least three episodes of wheezing and were considered to be at risk of developing asthma. The house-dust samples from the households whose children had asthma had significantly less endotoxin than the dust from healthy babies' homes. The more endotoxin they found in the house dust, the more immune activity was identified in the baby's blood (Lancet, 2000; 35: 1680–3).

Endotoxin is a component of the cell walls of certain bacteria that may trigger protective changes in an infant's immune system. Likewise, an Italian study found that respiratory allergy was less frequent in those heavily exposed to orofaecal and foodborne microbes, such as *Helicobacter pylori, Toxoplasma gondii* and hepatitis A virus. These pathogens, say the researchers, stimulate lymphoid tissue in the gut to produce chemicals which fight atopy. Moreover, these organisms need not cause disease to exert a protective effect (BMJ, 2000; 320: 412–7).

These findings call into question the concept of sterilisation, the use of antibacterial soaps and keeping children away from sick friends. However, the one proviso is that early exposure to bacteria is most likely to be health-enhancing when the child's health is well supported in other ways. This may include breastfeeding, since early exposure to cow's milk predisposes a child to atopy (BMJ, 1999; 319: 815–9), and a staged diet that does not introduce other known food allergens, such as cow's milk and wheat, too early in life.

Moulds, however, are potentially more dangerous. Relatives of mushrooms, some moulds can be as toxic as the most hazardous man-made chemicals.

To minimise your exposure to dust mites or mould:

◆ Keep the bedroom uncluttered and easy to clean.

◆ Regularly vacuum mattresses, box springs and pillows or, better still, encase them in airtight, zipped-up plastic covers.

◆ Before vacuuming, dust furniture, windowsills and crevices with a slightly damp cloth.

◆ Wash all bedding regularly in hot water (at least 130 degrees F) to kill dust mites.

◆ Choose Dacron or Orlon pillows and replace every two years.

◆ Remove as much carpeting as possible and replace with wood or vinyl flooring. To prevent mould, do not use carpets in bathrooms.

◆ Keep indoor humidity levels low (between 30 and 50 per cent) with either a dehumidifier or air conditioning.

◆ Use a vacuum cleaner with a HEPA (high-efficiency particulate air) or the newer ULPA (ultra-low penetration air) filter. Vacuuming won't suck up the dust mites themselves—they are great at clinging to fibres—but it will remove their droppings and decomposing body parts.

◆ Ventilate the bathroom daily to ensure that walls and curtains dry out completely.

◆ Clean baths, showers and curtains monthly with a 1:10 bleach-to-water solution to kill mould.

◆ Clean all air-filtering appliances regularly.

Smoking in the home

Passive smoking is a genuine threat and can increase the chances of heart disease, scientists have established in a major new study. They are calling for a ban on smoking in all public places and in homes where there are children.

People who are exposed to between one and 19 cigarettes a day increase their risk of heart disease by 1.23 times, and the risk rises to 1.31 times among those exposed to more than 20 cigarettes a day.

Although the increased risk seems small, it is important, say the researchers from Tulane University School of Public Health in New Orleans. Heart disease is the major killer in the West, accounting for 25 per cent of all deaths in the US. At least 100,000 lives in the US alone could be saved just by stopping smoking.

The researchers reviewed 18 studies into passive smoking and found that passive smokers had an overall risk of heart disease of 1.25 times compared with those not exposed to passive smoking.

It has been estimated that up to 43 per cent of children are exposed to cigarette smoke in their homes, childcare facilities and schools. "The only safe way to protect non-smokers from exposure to cigarette smoke is to eliminate this health hazard from public places and work-places, as well as from the home," they concluded (N Engl J Med, 1999; 340: 920–6).

Fears over halogen

Halogen is the latest trendy form of lighting, replacing track lighting as the darling of decorators, particularly in the kitchen and bathroom, and in public places such as restaurants and offices.

Halogen floor lamps, known as "halogen torchière lamps", are also extremely popular with students, providing a focused light far more intense than incandescent lighting. Halogen lamps are now a popular supplement to the poor fluorescent lighting of university dormitories.

These floor lights are built with an upright open shade containing a tubular halogen bulb and a thin glass guard over it to catch the pieces in case the bulb shatters.

The recent concern over halogen lamps has to do with their potential as a fire hazard—specifically, their propensity to ignite anything within reach that's combustible. In America, where an estimated 30 to 40 million torchière-style halogen floor lamps are currently in use, the lamps have been responsible for some 189 fires and at least 11 deaths since 1991, according to the Consumer Product Safety Commission (CPSC).

Jazz legend Lionel Hampton's home was destroyed when a halogen lamp caught fire. In Albany, New York, a halogen torchière lamp caused a fire which injured two young children. And one firefighter died in the blaze at an American university dormitory, which caught fire after a halogen lamp tipped over, igniting a hanging tapestry.

Unlike the common standard lamp, which employs incandescent bulbs of 60–100 watts, halogen floor lamps have bulbs with 300–500 watts, roughly five to 10 times more power. According to the CPSC, the lamps can generate ceiling temperatures of up to 1200 degrees.

The biggest problems tend to be caused when fabric is draped over the lamps or when they come in contact with curtains. Students in particular are notorious for draping clothing over lamps or leaving them in contact with fabric and other combustibles.

In the UK, several fires have started when overhead halogen lights were too close to objects in the room. One such fire occurred, says UK lighting specialist Christopher Wray, when a customer positioned one of his recessed low-voltage lights too near a kitchen cabinet.

Besides the problem of the intense heat generated by these lamps, there is also their propensity to tip over. "Our tests showed that it required only 17 ounces of force applied to the brass rung, which is 46 inches from the floor, to tip," says New York state fire administrator James Burns.

In the US, the CPSC, which is currently investigating 31 fires directly linked to halogen floor lamps, has the authority to look into product defects. Nevertheless, it doesn't set the standard for halogen lamps. That job falls to Underwriters Laboratories, an industry-funded group which sets a safety standard that is basically voluntary.

In the wake of all the fires, several American universities, such as the Rochester Institute of Technology in New York, have banned torchière-style halogen lamps. Other universities will only allow halogen lamps that meet certain standards into residence halls.

A number of bodies in the US and UK have modified the specifications for floor and ceiling halogen lighting. In America, after 5 February 1997, Underwriters Labs began requiring halogen floor lamps to undergo much tougher safety tests. However, one independent lab, Inchcape Testing Services, tested three varieties of the new floor lamps to see if the new safety features, such as lower wattage, made a difference to their potential to cause fires.

In the test, a lamp with a 300-watt bulb is left on for 15 minutes and a double layer of cheesecloth, which is highly inflammable, is draped over the top of the lamp. If it doesn't catch fire within seven hours, the lamp passes the test with flying colours. Nevertheless, in the recent Inchcape test, the first lamp caused the cheesecloth to go up in flames in 34 seconds; in the second, holes burned through the cheesecloth in 16 seconds and, in the third, the cheesecloth caught fire in 25 seconds—all this among lamps that had been recently redesigned to meet the new safety standards!

With halogen ceiling lamps, the main concern is not only what is under the lamps, but also what is above them; fires have started when the lamp is positioned near floor insulation, which also burns readily.

Less well known than the fire hazards are the problems of low-level radiation. UK's Alistair Philips at Powerwatch says that all halogen lights, whether free-standing or embedded in the ceiling, require low-voltage transformers (12, 24 or 48 volts) that are compatible with the voltage of the building (110 in the US; 240 in the UK). "Most of these transformers are 'cheap and cheerful' and usually quite crude," says

Philips. Consequently, transformers can create pools of strong magnetic fields three feet below, as well as above, the lights. This is worrying in a kitchen, where the maximum intensity of the field is close to where a tall adult would be standing, and even more so in the room above, which is often a bedroom where people could be sleeping inches away from the embedded ceiling lights of the floor below.

In one instance, Philips was called to test the electromagnetic fields around halogen ceiling lighting in the kitchen of a woman's farmhouse. Horrendous levels of EMFs were found in her daughter's bedroom, which lay directly above.

One way to reduce the EMFs generated by recessed halogen lighting is to have an electrician run all your halogen lights off one good-quality transformer that is placed, say, in a cupboard.

A final problem is caused by staring at these high-intensity bulbs for too long. The UK National Radiological Protection Board has produced a leaflet which says that prolonged staring at halogen bulbs can cause a condition in the eye not unlike macular degeneration, which affects central vision. This happened to Alistair Philips when he was filmed by a television production company for 15 minutes and asked to look into a camera with a halogen light whose diffuser was broken. Twelve hours later, a black patch appeared in the middle of one of his eyes, which was eventually diagnosed as a central serous retinopathy, a blister in the back of his retina. It took a full year before the condition cleared.

If you wish to have recessed lights, you can opt for the good old-fashioned incandescent variety, which are still better for you than fluorescent or halogen bulbs.

How to maintain a healthy house

Volatile organic compounds (VOCs)
♦ Check with the manufacturers of the products you are considering buying about their VOC outgassing potential.

- Allow new furniture, carpets and other furnishings to outgas outside the home, or ventilate for up to three days after installation.
- If buying a new home, check with the builder about whether he has used VOC-containing building materials.
- If the house appears to be particularly full of VOCs, do a 'bake-out'—that is, after the house is constructed, renovated or refurnished, heat it to a high temperature, usually 100 degrees F (38 degrees C). Open all the windows and run the ventilation system at full capacity. Repeat this process for two or three days. In theory, the high temperature will cause the materials in the house to release their chemicals more quickly, instead of over a period of months or years.
- Reduce VOCs by placing 'absorbers' in the room. These are made from substances such as zeolite or aluminium silicate, to which VOCs have been found to adhere.
- Limit the amount of carpet used in the home, and choose carpet with a latex-free backing. Do not glue carpet to the floor; use nailing or gripper strips instead.
- Avoid carpets treated with fungicides and permanent stain-resisting chemicals.
- When buying scatter-rugs, choose cotton-based materials.
- Use water-based paints and sealers, or seek out low-VOC paints.
- Choose solid wood cabinets and counters or, if they are made from composite-bonded materials, seal all the exposed surfaces with a water-based or low-toxicity sealant.
- Use a balanced mechanical ventilation system, such as a heat-recovery ventilator, to continuously expel indoor air and replace it with fresh outside air.

Combustion gases

- Try to site your gas or oil boiler/furnace in a dedicated room away from the living areas. If that's not practical, choose a boiler manufactured as a 'sealed combustion unit'.

- Cook with electricity as a first choice. If you have a gas range or hob, have the flames adjusted to burn correctly (they should burn blue; a yellow flame indicates incomplete combustion, which produces carbon monoxide).
- Choose a gas hob with an electronic igniter rather than a pilot light.
- Fit an extractor fan near the gas source. The fan should be vented to the outside; carbon-filtered recycling hoods simply recirculate the fumes back into the room.

Pesticides

- Choose 100-per-cent nylon carpets. Wool carpets are invariably treated with pesticides.
- Take your shoes off when you enter your house to avoid tracking in pesticides and other chemicals from the outdoors.

Electromagnetic fields (EMFs)

- Only use electric blankets to preheat a bed and turn if off once you are in bed.
- Heat waterbeds during the day, then turn off the heat in the evening before you go to bed.
- Avoid placing electrical clocks, fans, radios or answering machines too near your head when sleeping.
- Do not place a bed against a wall that is adjacent to a refrigerator, air-conditioning unit or fuse box.
- Do not site low-voltage lighting transformers near the bedroom.
- Consider installing a remote-control power breaker so that, at night, all power to the bedroom can be conveniently shut off.
- View TVs and computer screens from a reasonable distance.
- To minimise exposure to the high magnetic fields generated in kitchens, maintain a safe distance whenever possible from all electrical appliances, particularly microwaves (a distance of four feet is recommended). Despite their built-in safety features, leaks

of microwave radiation can occur. Do not use a microwave if it appears to be malfunctioning; treat even odd noises as suspicious.

Chapter 2
The truth about toxic toiletries

What could be more healthy than a refreshing body wash, a nourishing shampoo, a minty fresh toothpaste and a moisturising facial cream? Commercials, magazine advertisements and billboards bombard us with the message that soaping and scrubbing, exfoliating and moisturising can only be beneficial to our health.

Yet, the glossy images of well-scrubbed individuals hide a dangerous secret: too many of the toiletries and cosmetics we use are carcinogenic cocktails of hazardous waste. Most of the chemicals which go into our toiletries are no different from the harsh, toxic chemicals used in industry. Far from enhancing health, they pose a daily threat to it.

Propylene glycol (PG) is a wetting agent and solvent used in make-up, haircare products, deodorants and aftershave. It's also the main ingredient in antifreeze and brake fluid. Similarly, polyethylene glycol (PEG), a related agent found in most skin cleansers, is a caustic used to dissolve grease, the same substance you find in oven cleaners. Isopropyl, an alcohol used in hair-colouring rinses, hand lotions and fragrances, is also a solvent found in shellac.

Sodium lauryl sulphate (SLS)—used in toothpastes, shampoos and just about every personal cleansing solution—is a harsh detergent commonly used as an engine degreaser. Each of these ingredients readily penetrates the skin with potentially adverse consequences (see Chapter 3 on toothpastes).

Some of the most dangerous chemicals we put on our bodies in the name of beauty are hormone-disrupting, water-soluble ammonia derivatives. DEA (diethanolamine), TEA (triethanolamine) and MEA (monoethanolamine) are almost always in products that foam: bubble-baths, body washes, shampoos, soaps and facial cleansers.

They are used to thicken, wet, alkalise and clean. While they are irritating to the skin, eyes and respiratory tract (Rev Environ Contam Toxicol, 1997; 149: 1–86), DEA, MEA and TEA are not considered particularly toxic in themselves. However, once added to a product, these chemicals react readily with any nitrites present to form potentially carcinogenic nitrosamines, such as NDEA (N-nitrosodiethanolamine). Of the three, DEA and MEA pose the greatest risk to human health. Prolonged exposure to these can alter liver and kidney function (J Am Coll Toxicol, 1983; 2: 183–235) and even lead to cancer (Rev Environ Contam Toxicol, 1997; 149: 1–86).

Nitrites get into personal-care products in several ways. They can be added as anticorrosive agents, they can be released as a result of the degradation of other chemicals, specifically 2-nitro-1,3-propanediol (BNDP), or they can be present as contaminants in raw materials. Ingredients such as formaldehyde or formaldehyde-forming chemicals, or 2-bromo-2-nitropropane (also known as Bronopol), which can break down into formaldehyde, can also produce nitrosamines.

The long shelf life of most toiletries also increases the risk of creating a carcinogenic chemical reaction. Stored for a long time at elevated temperatures, nitrates will continue to form in a product, accelerated by the presence of other chemicals such as formaldehyde, paraformaldehyde, thiocyanate, nitrophenols and certain metal salts (Science, 1973; 181: 1245–6; J Nat Cancer Inst, 1977; 58: 409; Nature, 1977; 266: 657–8; Fd Cosmet Toxicol, 1983; 21: 607–13).

Inadequate and confusing labelling means that consumers may never know which products are most likely to be contaminated. However, in a recent US Food & Drug Administration (FDA) report, approximately 42 per cent of all cosmetics were contaminated with NDEA, with shampoos having the highest concentrations (National Toxicology Program, *Seventh Annual Report on Carcinogens*, Rockville, MD: US Department of Health and Human Services, 1994).

In Europe, where more safeguards are in place regarding nitrosating agents, the picture is somewhat better. In Germany, after the Federal

Health Office issued a request to eliminate all secondary amines (such as DEA) from cosmetics in 1987, a report confirmed that only 15 per cent of products tested were contaminated with NDEA (Eisenbrand G et al. in O'Neill IK et al., eds, *N-Nitrosoalkanolamines in Cosmetics*, Lyon: IARC, 1991).

Manufacturers insist that DEA and its relatives are safe in products designed for brief or discontinuous use, or those which wash off. However, there is evidence from both human and animal studies that NDEA is rapidly absorbed through the skin (J Natl Cancer Inst, 1981; 66: 125–7; Toxicol Lett, 1979; 4: 217–22). This argument also doesn't explain why these chemicals crop up regularly in body lotions and facial moisturisers which are, of course, meant to stay on the skin for long periods of time.

As far back as 1978, the International Agency for Research on Cancer (IARC) concluded that "although no epidemiological data were available, nitrosodiethanolamine should be regarded for practical purposes as if it were carcinogenic to humans" (IARC, 1978; 17: 77–82). This position was reaffirmed nearly 10 years later.

In the US in 1994, the National Toxicology Program similarly concluded in its *Seventh Annual Report on Carcinogens* that: "There is sufficient evidence for the carcinogenicity of N-nitrodiethanolamine in experimental animals." The report noted that, of more than 44 different animal species in which NDEA compounds have been tested, all have been susceptible (Lijinsky W, *Chemistry and Biology of N-Nitroso Compounds*, New York: Cambridge University Press, 1992). Humans are unlikely to be the single exception, said the paper.

The cosmetic industry's response to the problems of nitrosamine formation has been to put even more chemicals in their products in an attempt to slow or inhibit the formation of NDEA. These include ascorbic acid, sodium bisulphite, butylated hydroxyanisole (BHA), butylated hydroxytoluene (BHT), sodium ascorbate, ascorbyl palmitate and alpha-tocopherol. None has proved adequate to prevent nitrosamine formation (Cosmet Toiletr, 1994; 109: 53).

In 1996, the Cosmetics, Toiletries and Fragrance Association (*Cosmetic Ingredient Review Compendium*, Washington, DC, 1996) stated: "These chemicals [cocamide DEA, lauramide DEA, linoleamide DEA and oleamide DEA] should not be used as ingredients in cosmetic products containing nitrosating agents." Nevertheless, DEA, TEA and MEA continue to be widely used in a staggering variety of toiletries and cosmetics.

Something smells

Today, it is not enough to be clean, you must smell clean as well. Fragrance has become an important selling point for everything from fabric softeners to body washes. But, again, underneath the sweet smell of marketing success, there is the rank odour of potential disease. Almost without exception, modern perfumes are manufactured almost entirely from petrochemicals. More disturbingly, many of these chemicals are considered hazardous waste.

The nose is a chemical receptor. When you inhale a fragrance, you are breathing in the chemicals that make up that particular smell, and it is the particular combination of chemicals which causes the physiological, emotional and psychological reactions associated with fragrance.

In one study, researchers conducted a perfume challenge of people with asthma-like symptoms. Those who took part in the test inhaled perfume through their mouths (wearing a nasal plug) in two ways: first with a carbon-filter mask on and then directly. Both methods induced symptoms in allergic individuals and the carbon-filter mask provided no protection (Allergy, 1996; 51: 434–9).

In other words, the chemicals had an effect regardless of whether they were breathed through the nose. The sense of smell has a more direct connection to the brain than any other sense. Fragrances—no matter what their source—are able to breach the blood–brain barrier to gain direct access to the limbic system, which is, among other functions, the emotional switchboard of the brain.

Some observers feel that a violation of the limbic system by volatile chemicals plays an important role in multiple chemical sensitivity (Biol Psychiatry, 1992; 32: 218–42; Toxicol Ind Health, 1992; 8: 181–202).

You might think you are safe choosing those products which advertise 'natural' fragrances. Unfortunately, the difference between synthetic and natural is very limited, and all claims of 'natural' fragrances should be viewed with suspicion.

Consider the manufacturing process for rosewater: coal tar is heated to 230 degrees F and gives off toluene, which is treated with chlorine to produce benzyl chloride. Benzyl chloride is then treated with potassium cyanide to produce phenyl ethyl alcohol, the main ingredient of rosewater (Killheffer T, *Synthetic Perfumes*, Popular Science Encyclopaedia, vol 10: 229–34).

More than 5000 chemicals are used in fragrance manufacture (Ann Dermatol Venereol, 1986; 113: 31–41), 95 per cent of which are made from petroleum (report by the Committee on Science & Technology, *Neurotoxins: At Home and the Workplace*, US House of Representatives, No. 99-827). These include benzene derivatives, aldehydes and many other known toxins and sensitisers capable of causing cancer, birth defects, central nervous system disorders and allergic reactions. No agency regulates the fragrance industry, even though some observers believe that the chemicals in perfume are as damaging to health as tobacco smoke.

Fragrances can also be absorbed through the skin. The greater the emollient quality of the product you are using (such as skin creams), the greater the absorbency (J Appl Toxicol, 1997; 17: 153–8). When fragrance chemicals penetrate the skin, they can affect other organs. Some have been shown to cause discoloration of internal organs while others are toxic to the liver and kidneys. Still others accumulate in fatty tissue and are passed on to children through breastmilk.

Fragrances can be quick to saturate the blood, but slow to clear from the body. The chemical compound 1,8-cineole, also called eucalyptol (a main ingredient of eucalyptus oil), was shown to reach saturation point in the blood after only 18 minutes of inhalation. It takes nearly an hour and three-quarters, however, to clear it from the system once inhalation stops (Chem Senses, 1996; 21: 477–80). 1,8-Cineole, which is also present in tea tree oil, has been shown to cause severe central nervous symptoms in pets and small children, and can affect the liver and bone marrow. Limonene (D-limonene), a constituent of 1,8-cineole, is also a skin irritant that can cause contact dermatitis (Contact Derm, 1997; 36: 201–6) but only after it undergoes oxidation. This is why products that contain it should be kept in airtight containers and stored in the dark.

Although the UK government announced its intention to investigate the presence of nitro musks in commercial products in 1994, these chemicals still remain on sale. They were commonly used in laundry powders up until a few years ago and, although this use has been pretty much phased out, nitro musks continue to be used in soaps and other household and personal-hygiene products throughout Europe and the rest of the world. They are also present in our drinking water.

The nitro musk compounds musk tibetene, musk ambrette, musk moskene, musk ketone and musk xylene, as well as some non-nitro musks, are stored in fat tissue and are very slow to clear from the body (Chemosphere, 1996; 33: 17–8). In the meantime, they are carcinogenic.

In a recent survey in Germany, out of 72 human blood samples, 66 (or 91 per cent) contained significant amounts of nitro musks (J Chromatogr B Biomed Sci Appl, 1997; 693: 71–8). In a 1991 report by the US Environmental Protection Agency (EPA), toluene, one of the most common chemicals used in the preparation of perfumes, was found in every single fragrance sample collected by the agency. According to the report, the chemical was "most abundant in the auto parts store as well as the fragrance section of the department store". Toluene has been shown to cause cancer and nervous system damage, and is designated as a hazardous waste by the EPA.

An earlier report by the FDA of compounds used in cosmetics which most frequently involved adverse reactions identified five chemicals (alpha-terpineol, benzyl acetate, benzyl alcohol, limonene and linalool) that are among the 20 most commonly used in the products tested in the 1991 EPA report.

Most of the research into the adverse effects of fragrances centres around asthma. Perfume has long been known to be an environmental risk factor for asthma (Hum Biol, 1996; 68: 405–14). There is copious evidence that toluene can not only trigger asthma attacks, but can even bring on asthma in previously healthy people.

It is probably no coincidence that the incidence of asthma has increased in the past decade by 31 per cent. In the same period, deaths from asthma have also increased by 31 per cent. Some 72 per cent of asthma patients in one study had adverse reactions to perfume; their lung function dropped 18–58 per cent below baseline measurements (Am J Med, 1986; 80: 18–22). One Russian study concluded that childhood asthma was higher in areas where homes were situated near, among other places, perfume factories and busy roads, again pointing to the link between petroleum byproducts of all varieties and damaged health (Med Tr Prom Ekol, 1995; 5: 15–9).

We have learned from research into glue-sniffing that constantly inhaling volatile substances can cause permanent neurological and psychiatric damage. Children who inhale glue and solvents can become listless or violent, have poor concentration, and experience convulsions and even coma (Bull Narc, 1994; 46: 49–78). One of the main ingredients of these solvents is toluene. This begs the question: what is the difference between wearing perfume and sniffing glue?

Our exposure to fragrance doesn't end with perfume. Consider the daily exposure to other indoor pollutants, such as soaps, household cleaners, haircare products, laundry soaps, fabric softeners and even foods, and the total toxic load quickly begins to mount up.

Research into toxic toiletries tells us what we do not want to know, which may be why governments, manufacturers of personal-care products and consumers have stubbornly ignored the facts. For years, shelves full of make-up and toiletries have been our ticket to eternal youth and glamour. Yet, most of the products we use damage hair, skin and nails, making them look older and less healthy. They may even be putting us on the fast track to chronic illness and even death.

Toxic sanitary products

Toxic shock syndrome (TSS), identified in the US in 1980, is a potentially fatal severe infection of the blood, caused by the toxin TSST-1.

The toxin is produced by the otherwise benign *Staphylococcus aureus* bacteria, which is present in the warm moist parts of the human body, including the vagina. In nearly a third of the population, it tends to sit there and does no harm. Although we don't understand how the *Staph* bug is converted into this toxin, the majority of cases occur in young women, and are mainly caused by the use of tampons.

The current statistics are that one in 30,000 to one in a million women will contract TSS each year. In the US, the estimates are even higher: 17 cases a year of tampon-related TSS in every 100,000 women.

The symptoms of TSS are the body's wholesale effort to fight extreme poisoning—flu-like symptoms, sudden high temperature, dizziness, headache, sore throat, aching muscles, vomiting, diarrhoea, low blood pressure and a rash which resembles sunburn. The danger phase begins with a sudden drop in blood pressure and respiratory failure. If caught early enough, TSS can be treated quickly with antibiotics in hospital; the main problem is identifying the condition.

Left untreated, TSS can lead to kidney or respiratory failure or even heart attack. If you do survive, nearly every major organ may be affected. Victims typically lose their hair, fingernails and toenails, and often their concentration and memory, for as long as a year. Some women are left with liver and kidney problems or deafness and arthritis. Two-thirds of all cases occur the under-25, with those aged 15–19 most at risk, largely because their immune systems may not yet be fully developed.

In the UK, the Women's Environmental Network and the Alice Kilvert Tampon Alert (AKTA), an organisation run by the parents of Alice, a 15-year-old who died of TSS, have been at the forefront of campaigns to identify tampons as a significant health risk. Although medicine doesn't really know what it is in tampons that triggers the production of toxins, the AKTA says that the surface of the tampon may provide a place for bacteria to colonise. Although the longer the tampon is in place, the more bacteria can multiply, TSS has also occurred in women who change tampons regularly.

WEN notes that tampons absorb a goodly number of vaginal secretions along with menstrual blood. This can lead to vaginal dryness which, in turn, can damage vaginal walls, leading to peeling of the mucous membrane. WEN has gathered statistics showing that one-fifth of all tampon users suffer from 'micro-ulceration', which heals between periods, but with a long-term significance that is as yet unknown. It's thought that this micro-ulceration can lead to larger ulceration and increase bleeding. Up to three-quarters of all tampon users have some alteration to the mucous membrane of the vagina.

The greatest risk factor appears to be superabsorbent tampons, which appear to increase the risk of damage and ulceration. They also contain more rayon, which apparently changes the chemical environment of the vagina; fibres from tampons have been found in vaginal walls. By drying out and damaging the vaginal walls, the tampons may also make it easier for the bacterial toxins to make their way into the bloodstream.

Rayon, a synthetic fibre, is also potentially dangerous because the process of processing the eucalyptus woodpulp involves the use of chlorinated compounds, which creates dioxin as a byproduct, minute remnants of which remain in the fibre. The US Environmental Protection Agency has gone on record to say that dioxin causes cancer in humans and that there may be no safe level. Increasing evidence points to dioxin in sanitary products as a major cause of endometriosis.

Although the US mandates that absorbency rates be standardised and that the individual rates of every brand be printed on the outside packaging, these are not regulated in the UK. The best form of protection is to avoid tampons altogether, particularly if you are under 25. But, if you must use them, AKTA recommends that you use the lowest absorbency possible and a low fibre-loss brand, and change all your tampons every four to six hours.

In case you're feeling complacent about using sanitary towels, you might wish to see what the WEN has uncovered about these. Up until 1989, all sanitary towels were made from paper pulp entirely bleached with chlorine. This process not only produces dioxin, but hundreds of other organochlorine compounds, which wreak havoc with human health, making their way into our food and water supplies. However, now that the dangers of chlorine bleaching have been well publicised, some manufacturers have attempted to produce pulp bleached by alternative means.

The best means so far is a process called chemo thermo mechnical pulp (CTMP), which uses hydrogen peroxide and appears to be safer. Beware of methods called 'oxygen bleaching', which use a smaller percentage of chlorine gas and still release organochlorine compounds. British cotton-only tampons are bleached with hydrogen peroxide and sodium hypochlorite.

The new-style superthin towels pounced on by most manufacturers these days contain superabsorbent materials such as polyacrylate gels, the same substances used in disposable nappies. The initial studies which passed through the US and UK governments demonstrate that toxicity is low. However, we know that workers in plants which manufacture these gels suffer eye and lung damage. The bottom line is, we don't know the long-term dangers of these gels on women (or for that matter, on babies) or whether the plastic coverings used will be breeding grounds for illnesses like toxic shock syndrome.

Your safest bet is to stick with the older-style cotton towels, to avoid bleached varieties and perhaps to investigate the idea of reusable towelling, which are both good for you and the environment.

Chapter 3
Toothpastes: a close brush with poison

According to the US government and the Dental Association, you can't have too much of a good thing. We are bombarded from every direction by fluoride. Every last one of our dental products— from toothpaste, floss and toothpicks to fluoride drops or pills—now contains fluoride. This means that, with any and every means of dental hygiene, we are ingesting some (often unknown) amount of a substance that is more toxic than lead and almost as toxic as arsenic, and still used in some quarters to kill rats.

Although America acknowledges the potential toxicity of fluoride with warnings on labels, Britain has the flimsiest of controls over the claims made and warnings given concerning fluoride-containing products. There is no control over the daily consumption of fluoride and no limits on the amount an individual can purchase. If a person lives in an area with fluoridated water and uses fluoridated dental products, he could be taking in many times more fluoride than is considered acceptable. The World Health Organization warns that a chronic fluoride intake of 2.0–8.0 mg per day can lead to skeletal fluorosis, a debilitating and sometimes crippling bone disease.

The quantity of fluoride in toothpastes for children is even more of an issue as children, because of their smaller size, naturally can be poisoned with far lower levels. Dental fluorosis, where teeth are pitted and mottled because of too high an ingestion of fluoride, is well known in areas of water fluoridation.

The most damning aspect are the toothpastes on offer for children. Many of these use enticing flavours such as orange, bubble fruit and strawberry, a practice which only encourages them to swallow it. There is even a Barbie variety with a tutti-frutti flavour.

Toothpaste and all over-the-counter dental products are controlled under the cosmetics section of the Medicines Act and administered by the Cosmetic, Toiletry and Perfumery Association, a trade organisation which advises manufacturers on labelling for toothpaste, mouthwash and dental floss.

Manufacturers are allowed to include fluoride up to a concentration of 1500 parts per million (ppm) but, with no other information, this sort of statistic is meaningless to the average consumer. Fluoride tooth-pastes are also supposed to display a warning about unsupervised toothbrushing with a pea-sized amount of toothpaste to minimise swallowing by children under seven. They should also state that if you are using fluoride supplements (pills or drops), you should consult your dentist. Mouthwashes also often include fluoride, but there seems to be no labelling regulations to cover stating the amount of fluoride contained.

But these are only recommendations and not hard and fast rules. Since fluoride is not considered a drug either, manufacturers do not need to specify the amount of fluoride contained in their products or how much constitutes too high a daily dose. They also don't need to specify if they have a product licence or not as this is only required if some sort of therapeutic claim is made on the packaging.

To examine the levels of fluoride in dental products, mainly toothpastes, and the level of detail disclosed in the labelling on all products containing fluoride, holistic dentist Tony Lees conducted a survey of the products sold in most of the main outlets—supermarkets and major chemists—in a typical British city. He chose nearby Hereford and, in late April 2000, went undercover, purchasing one of each product at all the larger chain stores.

Lees was also interested in freedom of choice—whether the store in question offered any non-fluoridated alternatives, particularly for children. Finally, he wanted to see what types of warnings there were concerning accidental overdose, particularly in children.

His findings make a chilling commentary on the fact that toothpaste manufacturers, like most makers of toiletries, are basically allowed to provide the flimsiest of detail about their products.

The products

Boots the Chemists
Boots offered two fluoride-free toothpastes—its own brand and one by Kingfisher's. The rest of the toothpastes offered contained fluoride, and no children's toothpastes were free of the stuff. Boots also sells mouthwashes which contain fluoride, but offer no indication of percentages, and dental floss soaked in fluoride to the maximum level permitted of 1500 ppm.

At Boots, it is possible to purchase orange-flavoured fluoride tablets (Endekay Fluotabs, for those ages four and over) over the counter without prescription and with no verbal warnings given as to their usage. This product contains 200 tablets of 2.2 mg sodium fluoride, a level which certainly can cause fluoride intoxication, leading to dental fluorosis or worse in children.

It was particularly amazing to find a denture toothpaste specifically designed to clean dentures which, for some reason, contained 0.24 per cent sodium fluoride. Another inexplicable touch was the addition of the artificial sweetener saccharine. As it also contains bromochlorophene, a disinfectant, it is obviously not designed to be used like a normal toothpaste.

Boots also sells Theramed 2 in 1, a toothpaste and mouthwash combination. This product gives no indication of the amount of sodium fluoride it contains. It doesn't warn against unsupervised brushing for children or provide an advisory that anyone taking fluoride supplements should consult their dentist.

Safeway Stores
There was a limited choice of non-fluoride toothpastes available—only Sensodyne Sensitive tooth formula with strontium chloride (a heavy

metal used to alleviate the pain of age-related receding gums) and Euthymol, which contains antiseptics with a strong taste that children are not likely to find pleasant. There were no fluoride-free children's toothpastes on offer. Safeway also sells mouthwashes containing unspecified amounts of sodium fluoride.

Safeway's own brand, Savers toothpaste, contains a whopping 0.85 per cent sodium monofluorophosphate, which they haven't translated into parts per million on the packaging. (Our own calculation worked this out to be around 1118 ppm of fluoride or 140 mg in a 125-mL tube.) It makes a number of therapeutic claims, such as "helps prevent tooth decay and strengthens tooth enamel", but does not display a product licence (PL) number to substantiate them.

Another Safeway's own brand toothpaste is Oracle for Kids Strawberry Flavour Gel, with the word 'Kids' in giant letters on the tube. This strawberry-flavoured gel contains 0.4 per cent sodium monofluorophosphate (525 ppm or 39 mg in a 75-mL tube). The worry with a product with such a 'fun taste' as strawberry is that, although it might "encourage kids to clean their teeth", as the manufacturer says, it may also encourage them to swallow it.

Printed on the packaging was the following: "The performance claims made on Oracle for Kids Strawberry Flavour Gel are approved by the British Dental Health Foundation". The British Dental Health Foundation, for the uninitiated, is a self-appointed body consisting, in the main, of dental manufacturers plus some dentists.

Another worrying aspect of the packaging is that, although therapeutic claims are made, no PL number appears on the packaging.

The other brand that was available at Safeway was Signal Family Protection toothpaste. Also 'accredited' by the BDHF, this product contains 0.32 per cent sodium fluoride (1450 ppm or 145 mg in a 100-mL tube). This is enough to kill a child if a sufficiently large quantity is consumed. Not only is there no warning about the dangers associated with ingesting too much fluoride, but it also emphasises that "children love the great taste", implying that they may use it as much as possible. Despite claims about hardening tooth enamel, again no PL number is displayed.

Tesco Stores

Tesco's own brand, Total Care Kids, contains 0.4 per cent sodium monofluorophosphate, which appears to be a standard amount of fluoride used in kiddy toothpastes. Like most of the other products, there is no PL number displayed despite the therapeutic claims. It boasts that the product is "not tested on animals", which is a good thing for the laboratory monkeys and rats of the world as it contains around 526 ppm of fluoride (26 mg in a 50-mL tube) which can lead to mottling or cavitation of children's teeth if accidentally swallowed.

Tesco also sells Pearl Drops Smokers toothpaste. The manufacturer has not even bothered to give the percentage of fluoride contained in Pearl Drops, presumably because it figures that smokers are already engaging in slow-motion self-poisoning. Again, there is no warning about accidental overdosing and no PL number on display.

The only fluoride-free toothpastes available at Tesco were Euthymol and Sensodyne Sensitive. There were no fluoride-free brands for children.

Sainsbury's Supermarkets

This supermarket chain offers the widest choice. For those wishing to avoid fluoride, Sainsbury's carries both Kingfisher and its own-brand fluoride-free toothpaste. It also offers its own-brand 'low fluoride' Baby Tooth Gel, which contains 0.025 per cent sodium fluoride (110 ppm or 5.5 mg in a 50-mL tube). Although Sainsbury's labels this more fully than any other baby-tooth toothpaste in the survey, it still fails to match the poison warnings required by the US Food & Drug Administration on American brands of fluoridated toothpaste.

Sainsbury's also sells a Milk Teeth gel toothpaste for children aged 0–6, made by Macleans (SmithKline Beecham). This contains 525 ppm of sodium monofluorophosphate (26 mg in a 50-mL tube), a dosage more than five times higher than Sainbury's own-brand label. Macleans' product, available with a strawberry flavour, has the so-called accreditation of the British Dental Association, the UK dentists' trade union. Again, no PL number is displayed.

Lidl

Not only does this supermarket offer no fluoride-free toothpastes, but it sells some toothpastes with no amount specified for fluoride content. There are no child warnings, not even about minimising swallowing.

Dentalux Med 3 asserts on the packaging: "The combination of sodium monofluorophosphate and sodium fluoride strengthens the gums and therefore helps to protect the teeth from decay." This is an untenable therapeutic claim as there is no evidence that sodium fluoride strengthens the gums. Furthermore, this toothpaste offers no advice on children's toothbrushing or about the quantities of fluoride added to the toothpaste. Needless to say, there is no PL number given.

Lidl's DentaLux 2 in 1, a mouthwash and toothpaste combination, doesn't specify the levels of fluoride it contains. There are also no swallowing warnings, no brushing advice and again, despite therapeutic claims, no PL number on the packaging.

Lidl's Unodent Plus toothpaste contains 1450 ppm of fluoride, which is an extremely poisonous level—145 mg in a 100-mL tube—enough to kill a child if ingested in quantity. Nevertheless, there are no warnings about the use of this product by children.

Dentalux in family size (125 mL) makes the claim that "the latest research shows that the active ingredients in Dentalux help to prevent tooth decay and gum disease". The product contains "Olafluor", a proprietary combination of "bis(hydroxyethyl) aminopropyl-N-hydroxyethyl octadecyclamin dihydrofluoride". Whatever this is—and we've never heard of it before—it is included in an unspecified quantity. There are no warnings whatsoever about accidental swallowing by children under seven, and no advisory about using a pea-sized amount of paste to minimise swallowing. No PL number is displayed.

Kwik Save Stores (owned by Somerfield Stores)

Kwik Save offered no choice of any fluoride-free toothpastes. Somerfield's Freshmint fluoride toothpaste contains 0.22 per cent sodium fluoride (995 ppm or 100 mg in a 100-mL tube), enough to seriously injure a child.

Deciphering the label: What does it all mean?

Fluoride toothpastes in the US are required to show a poison label. The American consumer is warned about swallowing the product and a toll-free Poisons Bureau telephone number is given in case the toothpaste is accidentally swallowed.

In the UK, the labelling of fluoride toothpaste and other fluoridated products is nothing short of haphazard. Fluorides in dental over-the-counter products carry a potent risk of acute and chronic fluoride poisoning. There is no question that easy availability of these products and the poor labelling pose a serious threat to health, particularly in children.

In our survey, labelling information was inconsistent. Some companies listed the amount of fluoride in ppm and some in percentages, some in both and some not at all. The British Dental Association (BDA) has recommended that all toothpastes should list their fluoride content in ppm as this is the easiest way to make the total amount of fluoride in any given product clear.

Choosing a low ppm toothpaste for your child is essential to limit the amount of fluoride ingested. Not long ago, researchers in Manchester set out to determine how much fluoride was being retained in children's mouths after brushing with toothpastes with 400 to 1450 ppm. The average amount of fluoride ingested per brushing was 0.42 mg when using the 1450 ppm toothpaste and 0.10 mg when using the 400 ppm one. If the 400 ppm toothpaste is used twice daily, a child of average weight would not ingest in excess of 0.05 mg/kg body weight (considered a 'safe' level)—but using the 1450 ppm toothpaste would certainly exceed this level (Br Dent J, 1999; 186: 460–2).

Unfortunately, not all toothpaste tubes show fluoride content in ppm. Some manufacturers include percentages, which are not helpful because they do not refer directly to the amount of fluoride in the tube. In fact, these percentages refer to the chemical compound of which fluoride is a part. Sodium fluoride, for example, is a compound containing sodium and fluoride whereas sodium monofluorophosphate comprises sodium, fluoride and phosphate.

To figure out the amount of fluoride in your toothpaste, you need to look for the ppm. If your toothpaste tube only lists percentages, there is a way to translate this to arrive at the amount of fluoride in the tube. The following chart will help you work out the approximate ppm of your toothpaste:

ppm	Sodium fluoride	Sodium monofluorophosphate
1500	0.32 per cent	1.14 per cent
1000	0.22 per cent	0.76 per cent
500	0.11 per cent	0.38 per cent

To find out how many milligrammes (mg) of fluoride are in the tube, divide the ppm by 1000, then multiply that by the number of millilitres (mL) in the tube. Thus, 1500 ppm $\div$ 1000 $\times$ 125 mL = 87.5 mg

As a rough guide, in each 100-mL tube of toothpaste, there are the following amounts of fluoride:

ppm	mg/100 mL
1500	150
1000	100
500	50

Why is there so much fluoride in toothpaste and mouthwash? Because these products are meant to be rinsed out of the mouth, so it is thought that we only retain a proportion of the fluoride. That idea, of course, is only relevant to the laboratory. In the real world, children don't always spit toothpaste out. They may be too young to control their swallowing, or it may simply be that sweet flavours and pretty colours make toothpaste as appealing as candy to swallow.

Also, fluoride can be unstable. Depending on the formulation, the amount of fluoride in toothpaste can deteriorate rapidly. When sodium fluoride is combined with aluminium and/or calcium containing abrasives, the mixture will lose 60–90 per cent of the added fluoride after one week's storage at room temperature (J Dent, 1989; 17: 47–54). Manufacturers may add more of it to overcome this problem.

Sodium lauryl sulphate and propylene glycol

Fluoride isn't the only ingredient that can damage your health. Sodium lauryl sulphate (SLS) and propylene glycol are also routinely included in the majority of toothpastes. These chemicals are also extremely hazardous.

SLS is a harsh detergent and wetting agent used in garage floor cleaners, engine degreasers and automobile cleaning products. According to the Journal of the American College of Toxicology (vol 2, no 7, 1983), it's a well-known skin irritant that is rapidly absorbed and retained in the eyes, brain, heart and liver, and has been linked to cataract formation and poor eye development in children.

Carcinogenic nitrates can also form in the manufacturing of SLS or by its interreaction with other nitrogen-bearing ingredients. US Material Safety Data Sheets warn: "DO NOT GET IN EYES, ON SKIN, ON CLOTHING. AVOID PROLONGED OR REPEATED EXPOSURE."

Propylene glycol is a form of mineral oil found in automatic brake and hydraulic fluid, and industrial antifreeze. In personal-care products, it acts as a humectant, so it is included in toothpaste to prevent the paste from drying up when the cap is left off. The *Safety Data Sheets* warn users to avoid skin contact, as this strong skin irritant can cause liver abnormalities and kidney damage.

To obtain dental care products that are totally free of carcinogens and other toxins, and approved by both the Cancer Prevention Coalition and the Children's Health Environmental Coalition, the safest source of which we are aware is an American company called Neways International. This company makes a wide range of personal-care, household-care and nutritional products which are so safe and effective that they have been recommended by Philip Day in his new book *Cancer: Why We're Still Dying to Know the Truth* (Credence; ISBN 0-955535012-4-8).

It's possible to register as a Neways wholesale customer for a one-off fee of only £10. Neways' UK office can be located on info@neways.co.uk or tel: 0180 861 764.

Chapter 4
Killer cosmetics

Every time you put on make-up, you lather your face with a deadly cocktail of carcinogens, preservatives, mutagens, allergens, toxic heavy metals and other poisons that slip through the loose regulatory net.

Many women think that make-up is just a bit of harmless feel-good fun and that the make-up they put on their faces each day—and wear for long hours at a time—is just a benign enhancement to beauty.

Yet, by the time a woman has made-up her face, she will have covered her skin with carcinogens and preservatives, mutagens (substances that cause genetic mutations), allergens, central nervous system disruptors, toxic heavy metals and poisons.

Make-up is a particularly insidious form of pollution because its chemical ingredients enter the body through multiple routes. We can swallow, inhale and absorb them through the skin as well as through the mucous membranes of the eyes, mouth and nose.

In addition, cosmetics commonly contain moisturisers in the form of wetting agents (such as propylene glycol) and humectants (such as glycerine) which, while relatively harmless in themselves, increase the skin's permeability, thus allowing more of these toxic ingredients to be absorbed into the body (Walters KA, Hadgraft J, eds, *Pharmaceutical Skin Penetration Enhancement*, New York: Marcel Dekker, 1993; Hseih DS, ed, *Drug Permeation Enhancement: Theory and Applications*, New York: Marcel Dekker, 1994).

Many assume that the government oversees the safety and efficacy of cosmetics. But make-up manufacturers are not required by the US Food & Drug Administration (FDA) or the UK Department of Trade and Industry (DTI) to demonstrate that their products are either safe or effective. What regulations there are do little to protect the consumer (Erickson K, Epstein SS, *Drop Dead Gorgeous*, New York: Contemporary Books, 2002).

While more than 3000 ingredients are approved for cosmetics use in Europe, many more find their way into products via loopholes in the law—such as those that allow traces of banned substances if they cannot reasonably be removed during or after manufacture. The only way to know if a cosmetic is safe is to trawl through its ingredients. Unfortunately, manufacturers are inconsistent in listing these. Some print them on the container or on peelaway labels on the underside of the product. Others list them on the box (which is often thrown away without a glance) or just don't list them at all as it's not required by law. So, it's very difficult for consumers to make good decisions about what products are safe.

Allergies and more

While generally underreported, cosmetic makers know that 10–30 per cent of adults experience skin reactions (Contact Derm, 1988; 19: 195–201). The worst reactions are due to fragrances and preservatives (Contact Derm, 1987; 17: 26–34; Contact Derm, 1984; 11: 265–7). In one study, 80 per cent of those who developed make-up reactions had had no prior skin problems (Contact Derm, 1999; 40: 310–5).

European studies show that the fragrance part of a product accounts for as much as 15 per cent of all allergic reactions in those with eczema (Contact Derm, 1997; 36: 57–86; Ned Tijdschr Geneeskd, 1997; 141: 571–4). Although synthetic fragrances are most commonly implicated, emerging evidence suggests that natural fragrances may also cause allergic reactions (J Invest Dermatol, 2000; 115: 129–30).

Fragrance is a particularly thorny issue for consumers as most of us will never know which fragrance chemicals are in the products we use. Manufacturers are allowed to list them under the catch-all heading of 'fragrance', which belies the often hundreds of different ingredients involved in a single scent (even the simplest use 40–50 ingredients). Most of these are neurotoxic chemicals associated with central nervous system (CNS) disorders such as multiple sclerosis, Alzheimer's and Parkinson's diseases, and sudden infant death syndrome. Many have even been labelled 'toxic waste' by the FDA.

Adult cosmetics are not the only problem. Play make-up and perfumes for children often contain unacceptably high levels of these substances (Contact Derm, 1999; 41: 84–8). According to the US Environmental Protection Agency report *Health Hazard Information* (EPA, 1991), the 20 most common fragrance ingredients constitute a toxic soup that no thinking person would wish to be exposed to. Of these chemicals, seven—1,8-cineole, beta-citronellol, beta-myrcene, nerol, ocimene, beta-phenethyl alcohol and alpha-terpinolene—are completely lacking in safety data. As for the rest:

◆ **Acetone** is on the hazardous waste lists of several government agencies. It is a CNS depressant which can cause dryness of the mouth and throat, dizziness, nausea, lack of coordination, slurred speech, drowsiness and, in severe exposures, coma.

◆ **Benzaldehyde** acts as a local anaesthetic and CNS depressant, and can cause irritation to the mouth, throat, eyes, skin, lungs and GI tract, causing nausea and abdominal pain. It can also cause kidney damage.

◆ **Benzyl acetate** is an environmental pollutant and potential carcinogen that has been linked to pancreatic cancer. Its vapours are irritating to the eyes and respiratory airways, and it can also be absorbed through the skin, causing systemic effects.

◆ **Benzyl alcohol** is irritating to the upper respiratory tract, and can cause headaches, nausea, vomiting, dizziness, blood pressure falls, CNS depression and even death due to respiratory failure.

◆ **Camphor** is a local irritant and CNS stimulant that is readily absorbed by body tissues. Inhalation can irritate the eyes, nose and throat, and cause dizziness, confusion, nausea, muscle twitches and convulsions.

◆ **Ethanol** is on the EPA hazardous waste list as it causes CNS disorders, and irritates the eyes and upper respiratory tract even at low concentrations. Inhalation of its vapours has the same effect as ingestion, involving an initial stimulatory effect followed by drowsiness, impaired vision, loss of muscle coordination and stupor.

◆ **Ethyl acetate** is on the EPA hazardous waste list and is a narcotic that is irritating to the eyes and respiratory tract. It can cause headache and stupor, and has a defatting effect on skin which may lead to drying and cracking. In extreme cases, it may cause damage to the liver and kidneys, and anaemia with high white cell counts.

◆ **Limonene** is a carcinogen as well as a skin and eye irritant and allergen.

◆ **Linalool** is a narcotic known to cause CNS disorders. It may lead to sometimes fatal respiratory disturbances, poor muscle coordination and reflexes, and depression. Animal tests show that it may also affect the heart.

◆ **Methylene chloride** was banned by the FDA in 1988, but no enforcement is possible due to trade-secret laws protecting the chemical fragrance industry. Occupying the hazardous waste lists of several government agencies, it is a carcinogen and CNS disruptor that is absorbed by and stored in body fat; it metabolises to carbon monoxide, reducing the amount of oxygen in the blood. Other adverse effects include headache, giddiness, stupor, irritability, fatigue and tingling in the limbs.

- **alpha-Pinene** is a skin-sensitising agent that is damaging to the immune system.

- **gamma-Terpinene** causes asthma and CNS disorders.

- **alpha-Terpineol** is highly irritating to mucous membranes. Breathed into the lungs, it can lead to pneumonitis or even fatal water retention. It can also cause nervous excitement, loss of muscle coordination, low body temperature, CNS and respiratory depression, and headache. Scientific data warn against its repeated or prolonged skin contact.

The most commonly used cosmetic preservatives are alkyl hydroxy benzoates—methylparaben, ethylparaben, butylparaben and propyl-paraben—either alone or, more often, in combination. Parabens are well recognised as skin sensitisers (causing skin reactions), and the UK's Brunel University has found parabens to be oestrogen mimics as well (Toxicol Appl Pharmacol, 1998; 153: 12–9). Lab tests showed that each type of paraben had a different oestrogenic potency, with methylparaben being the least potent.

Kathon CG (mainly methylisochlorothiazolinone and methylchloro-thiazolinone) is the next most commonly used preservative in cos-metics, and is also a common allergen (Contact Derm, 1986; 14: 155–7). A recent study from the University of Texas found that Kathon CG is capable of causing genetic mutations (Environ Mol Mutagen, 1996; 28: 127–32).

Mercury rising

Many of us laugh at the obviously dangerous fashions of the past, like painting of the face white with lead, and believe that today's cosmetics represent a huge step forward in both beauty and safety. But the National Report on Human Exposure to Environmental Chemicals, compiled by the US Centers for Disease Control (CDC) in 2001, noted that, while levels of lead in human tissues appear to be declining, there has been a rise in, among other things, levels of mercury.

Mercury-containing ingredients, such as phenylmercuric acetate, are common in cosmetics. Indeed, the same preservative is found in vaccines, toiletries such as soap-free cleansers, antiseptic sprays, make-up remover, eye moisturisers and mascara. These refer to mercury by one of its many synonyms—Mercurochrome, Merthiolate, sodium ethylmercurithiosalicylate, thimerosalate, thiomerosal, merzonin, mertorgan, ethyl (2-mercaptobenzoate-S) or merfamin—which aren't readily identifiable as mercury (see *The Merck Index*, 12th edn, 1996, p 1590, for the complete list).

Heavy metals also get into cosmetics in other ways. Often, they are contaminants in pigments and talc. One Finnish study looked at 88 brands of eyeshadow for the presence of lead, cobalt, nickel, chromium and arsenic, and found that 66 (75 per cent) of the products had more than 5 ppm (parts per million) of at least one of these elements. The highest levels of cobalt and nickel were 41 ppm and 49 ppm, respectively—enough to cause an allergic reaction in those who are sensitive (Contact Derm, 2000; 42: 5–10).

In this instance, the elements in these cosmetics were impurities rather than actual listed ingredients, a problem shared by many cosmetics. While the researchers felt that, in most cases, the levels were not enough to cause allergic reactions, a UK study found that chronic exposure to very low levels of arsenic—lower than those in the Finnish study—could disrupt hormone levels (Environ Health Perspect, 2001; 109: 5–10).

Sunscreen hype

Sunscreens are also easily absorbed through the skin into the blood-stream, the effects of which are still unknown (Lancet, 1997; 350: 863–4).

Screening chemicals in suncreams, lipsticks and other cosmetics have been revealed by Swiss researchers to be hormone-disrupting chemicals. In lab tests of six common chemicals—benzophenone-3,4-methylbenzylidene camphor (4-MBC), homoslate, octylmethoxy-cinnamate, octyldimethyl-PABA and butylmethoxydibenzoylmethane (B-MDM)—all but B-MDM acted like oestrogen in making cancer cells grow more rapidly. Japanese research has also confirmed the oestrogenic potential of sunscreens (Toxicology, 2000; 156: 27–36).

Increasing exposure to endocrine disrupters is associated with a wide range of women's problems, such as breast cancer, cystic ovaries and endometriosis. These agents are also associated with problems in men, such as prostate and testicular cancers, and poor semen quality (Sci Total Environ, 1997; 205: 97–106; BMJ, 2001; 323: 1317–8).

Colours

Most of us avoid foods that contain artificial colours. Yet, every day, women paint their faces with a range of artificial colours known to cause health problems.

Artificial colours may be carcinogens (such as all coal-tar dyes) whereas others may contain hidden carcinogenic impurities. While use of a single make-up product may be 'safe', your total daily exposure to coloured products—in soap, shampoo, conditioner, shaving cream, toothpaste, deodorant, juices, cereals, pastries, coffee, creamer, even vitamins—may add up to an unacceptable risk.

Checking for harmful dyes in cosmetics is a complex business, made more difficult by the fact that, in Europe, these colours are usually listed by their INCI (International Nomenclature for Cosmetic Ingredients) numbers—usually 'CI' followed by five numbers—which is different again from the name given to the same ingredient when used as a food colouring—usually an 'E' followed by a number. The only consistent numbers used throughout the world is the CAS (Chemical Abstract Registry) number (see table, p 60).

New colours are being developed all the time, but not with an eye on safety. FD&C red 40 (allura red, CI16035, CAS 25956-17-6, or E129) is a popular addition to eyeshadow. It has been approved and used since 1994 despite the fact that all safety tests were funded and carried out by the manufacturer. The US National Cancer Institute reports that p-credine, a chemical used in making FD&C red 40, is a carcinogen.

List of killer colours

Most cosmetic colours are considered capable of causing cancer—such as D&C reds 2, 3, 4, 10, 17 and 23; and FD&C red 10 and blue 4—but can be regularly found in many cosmetics that are routinely sold in Europe and the US.

Common name	US	Europe	E no	CAS
Pigment red 53 sodium salt	D&C red 8	CI15585	–	2092-56-0
Pigment red 53 barium salt	D&C red 9	CI15585	–	5160-02-1
Rhodamine B	D&C red 19	CI45170	–	
Alizarine cyanine green F	D&C green 5	CI61570	–	4403-90-1
Pigment orange 5	D&C orange 17	CI12075	–	
CI Disperse Blue 1	Disperse Blue 1	CI64500	–	2475-45-8
CI Disperse Yellow 3	Disperse Yellow 3	CI3/1185	–	2832-40-8
Fast green FCF	FD&C green 3	CI42053	–	2353-45-9
Ponceau SX	FD&C red 4	CI14700	–	4548-53-2
Tartrazine	FD&C yellow 5	CI19140	E102	1934-21-0
Sunset yellow	FD&C yellow 6	CI15985	E110	2781-94-0
Brilliant blue FCF	FD&C blue 1	CI42090	E133	3844-45-9
Indigo carmine	FD&C blue 2	CI73015	E132	860-22-0

Long-term dangers

A 75-year-old woman who develops cancer would not assume that her lifetime use of cosmetics was a contributing factor. But increasingly, it appears that cosmetics contribute significantly to the total toxic load, leading to diseases such as cancer, CNS disorders and autoimmune diseases.

Liquid formulas, such as make-up foundations, often contain carcinogenic nitrosamines, usually from combining formaldehyde-releasing agents such as 2-bromo-2-nitropropane-1,3 diol or quaternium-15 and amines such as triethanolamine. The longer the product is on the shelf, the higher the risk of nitrosamine formation.

Most types of make-up also contain the preservative butylhydroxyanisole (BHA), a chemical that is easily absorbed into the skin and designated a carcinogen by the US National Toxicology Program (NTP). Mascara—especially those that claim to extend your lashes—can contain any number of carcinogenic plasticisers like polyurethane.

Another common ingredient is silica, usually touted as a natural skin-enhancing mineral in spite of the fact that cosmetic silica is synthesised in the lab. Two years ago, crystalline silica (crystalline quartz; also found in cat litter and scouring powders) was added to the NTP list of carcinogens (*9th Report on Carcinogens*, NTP, May 2000). While silica may be used in any cosmetic, the most risky are those that are easily inhaled, such as face powder and eyeshadow. The silica commonly used in cosmetics may be contaminated with the carcinogenic crystalline form, but it is impossible to tell which silica-containing products are contaminated. Using any silica-containing product is simply playing cosmetic Russian roulette.

Most make-up—even powder formulations—contain mineral oil to bind the ingredients together, and to provide a base for liquid formulas and lipsticks. Mineral oils were first recognised as carcinogens in 1987. Listed as 'parafinnum liquidim' (the stuff that baby oil is made from) or 'petrolatum' (petroleum jelly), these highly refined oils have a chequered history. Mineral oils are also thought to increase skin photosensitivity, making it more prone to sun damage.

As the mineral oils in cosmetics are highly refined, scientists can't tell exactly how dangerous they are to humans. The thinner the oil (as in parafinnum liquidim), the riskier it is thought to be because of the high levels of volatile hydrocarbons thin oils contain. The National Toxicology Program's carcinogens report notes that analyses of mineral oils used for medicinal and cosmetic purposes reveal the presence of several carcinogenic hydrocarbons known as polycyclic aromatic hydrocarbons. These include benzo[b]fluoranthene, benzo-[k]fluoranthene and benzo[a]pyrene.

The dangers of mineral oils were underscored recently when, in 2001, the US Consumer Product Safety Commission enacted a new law requiring safety caps for all toiletries containing thin mineral oils (parafinnum liquidium), including baby oils and suntan lotions.

The move came after a 16-month-old baby in California died after ingesting and inhaling baby oil. The commission noted that during the years 1997–1999, 64,000 children under five were brought to emergency rooms with suspected ingestion or inhalation of mineral oil hydrocarbons.

The move was vigorously opposed by the US Cosmetic, Toiletry and Fragrance Association, which argued that only automotive and household chemicals should be forced to have safety caps put on their products. But this argument ignores the fact that the ingredients in toiletries and cosmetics are often exactly the same as those used by the automotive industry and in household cleaners.

When considering the things that influence good health, most of us recognise that environment has an increasingly strong influence on our day-to-day health. We understand pollution from factories and cars, in our water and on the food we eat. But there is still a lack of awareness of the contributory effects of household and personal-care products, especially cosmetics. Women who wear make-up are exposing themselves for most of the day, and often seven days a week, to an ugly cocktail of allergens, carcinogens, and hormone and CNS disruptors - all in the name of beauty.

Cancer-causing ingredients

Cosmetics can contain frank carcinogens, those that are inherently carcinogenic, or hidden carcinogens, those that become carcinogenic under certain circumstances, such as when mixed, or contaminated by frank carcinogens (Epstein SS, *Unreasonable Risk, Environmental Toxicology*, 2001). The most common of these are:

Benzyl acetate*
Butylated hydroxyanisole (BHA)
Butylated hydroxytoluene (BHT)
Butyl benzylphthalate
Crystalline silica
Crystalline silica (inhaled)
Diaminophenol
Diethanolamine (DEA)
Dioctyl adipate
Ethyl alcohol*
Fluoride*
Formaldehyde
Glutaral
Hydroquinone
Methylene chloride
Nitrophenylenediamine
Phenyl-p-phenylenediamine
p-Phenylenediamine* (following oxidation)
Polyvinyl pyrrolidone (PVP)
Pyrocatechol
Saccharin
Talc
Titanium dioxide*

Suspected carcinogens, though evidence is limited

Choose your make-up carefully

When it comes to make-up, it may be a case of choosing your poison carefully. If your lifestyle is relatively toxin-free, the use of well-chosen make-up may not add much to your total toxic load.

When you do buy or use cosmetics, follow these simple guidelines to help you choose the safest ones:

◆ *Start on the inside.* Beauty really does come from within. It starts with a nutritious diet, adequate rest and periodic stress-free breaks. Without these basics, no make-up will make you look beautiful.

◆ *Read the label.* Don't rely on claims of 'all natural', 'organic' or 'cruelty-free'. These claims are meaningless. The true story of the product can only be found in the list of ingredients. Once you have identified an ingredient(s) that you wish to avoid, write the name(s) on a card or list to take with you whenever you shop. Also, price is no guarantee of safety or quality. Sometimes, the cheaper brands use fewer toxic ingredients—but only the label will tell you for sure.

◆ *But don't put too much faith in the label.* And don't just buy a product because it was safe the last time you looked. By the time you replace your eyeshadow or lipstick, it may be using completely different ingredients. Manufacturers are continually reformulating their products, often according to what ingredients are available and least expensive at the time. In addition, many ingredients labels, such as those on eyeshadows and lipsticks, list the colours for the entire range rather than the specific item you're buying. Some products say 'may include . . .' or use '+/-' before a list of ingredients, rendering it impossible to make sensible choices about safety.

◆ *Avoid cosmetics that are pearly, glittery, opalescent or frosted.* These are among the most dangerous because, to achieve these effects, the manufacturers add ingredients such as pure aluminium, mica and even fish scales. Used near the eye, these particles can flake off and cause corneal damage. Ingested aluminium is linked to Alzheimer's disease. So, stick to matte colours, blot well and shine up your lips with a over- or undercoat of shea butter or natural oils.

◆ *Choose lip gloss (which has a lower volume of colour ingredients) over lipstick for everyday wear, but be aware.* Conventional lip glosses contain less colour, but are high in phenol, a poisonous substance that is easily absorbed into the delicate tissue of the lips (aided by petrolatum, a petroleum-derived moisturiser, along with other wetting agents). Phenol ingestion can cause nausea, vomiting, convulsions, paralysis, respiratory collapse and even death. Minute amounts are linked with skin rash, swelling, pimples and hives.

◆ *Seek 'safe' colours.* In cosmetics terms, a number beginning with 'CI75 . . .' is considered a 'natural' colourant, even though some are highly synthesised. Anything else may be considered suspect. Those beginning with 'CI77 . . .' are inorganic substances used as colourings (such as iron oxides, natural carbon, and the more toxic aluminium and barium sulphates).

◆ *Avoid all perfumed cosmetics, especially those lip products which taste sweet.* Often, these use saccharin (a suspected carcinogen) and phthalic anhydride (made from another suspected carcinogen, naphthalene), an irritant which can cause headaches, nausea, vomiting, diarrhoea and confusion. It has also been linked to kidney and brain damage in infants—all the more remarkable as it is commonly used in 'play' and 'fun' make-up aimed at young girls.

◆ *Choose products that don't contain sunscreens.* Chances are, you mostly wear your make-up indoors anyway. Don't be fooled by claims of natural sunscreens. There's no such thing. The only effective sunscreens are synthetic chemicals that merely add to your toxic burden.

◆ *If you don't need to wear make-up, don't.* Many women wear make-up for the most trivial occasions—to go shopping for groceries, on the weekend at home or for taking a walk in the park. Get out of the habit. Get used to the way you look without make-up, and give your skin and body a break. If you simply must put something on your face, stick to the basics—a swipe of carefully chosen mascara and a bit of lipstick or lip gloss is fine for everyday use.

Ingredients to avoid

When selecting kinder cosmetics and toiletries, choose products which do not have any of the following ingredients:

◆ **DEA, MEA, TEA.** Can cause allergic reactions, irritate the eyes, and dry the hair and skin. Can be carcinogenic, especially to kidney and liver.

◆ **Petrolatum, also known as mineral oil jelly, liquid Vaseline, paraffinum liquidum and baby oil.** Can cause photosensitivity and strips the natural oils from the skin, causing chapping and dryness, and also premature ageing. Prevents elimination of toxins. Can cause acne and other disorders.

◆ **Imidazolidinyl urea and DMDM hydantoin.** These formaldehyde-forming preservatives can cause joint pain, allergies, depression, headaches, chest pain, chronic fatigue, dizziness, insomnia and asthma. Can also weaken the immune system and even cause cancer. Found in skin, body and hair products, antiperspirants and nail polish.

- **Alcohol, or isopropyl.** A poisonous solvent and denaturant (altering the structure of other chemicals). Found in hair colour rinses, body rubs, hand lotions, aftershave lotions and fragrances. Can cause nausea, vomiting, headaches, flushing and depression. Also, dries skin and hair, creating cracks and fissures in the skin which encourage bacterial growth.

- **Sodium lauryl sulphate (SLS).** Found in shampoos, hair conditioners, toothpastes and body washes. A strong detergent which can cause eye irritation, permanent damage to the eyes, especially in children, skin rashes, hair loss, flaking skin and mouth ulceration. When combined with other ingredients, can form nitrosamines, which are carcinogenic. Easily penetrates the skin and able to lodge itself in the heart, lungs, liver and brain.

- **PVP/VA copolymer.** A petroleum-based ingredient used in hairsprays.

- **Padimate-O, also known as octyl dimethyl, PABA.** Found mostly in sunscreens. Like DEA, a nitrosamine-forming agent. There is concern that the energy absorbed by this sunscreen is then turned into free radicals, which may actually increase the risk of skin cancer.

- **Methyl, propyl, butyl and ethyl parabens.** Used to extend a product's shelf life and inhibit microbial growth. Highly toxic. Can cause rashes and other allergic reactions.

Synthetic colours

- **Coal-tar dyes.** Generally labelled as 'FD&C' or 'D&C', followed by a number. Carcinogenic.

◆ **Talc**. Found in baby powders, face powders and body powders as well as on contraceptives such as condoms. A known carcinogen. A major cause of ovarian cancer when used in the genital area. Can also lodge in the lungs, causing respiratory disorders.

◆ **Fragrance.** Usually petroleum-based. Can cause headaches, dizziness, rashes, respiratory problems, vomiting, skin irritation and multiple chemical sensitivity.

Chapter 5
Multiple chemical sensitivity

A n 'environmental illness' is a genuine condition with a number of recognisable symptoms that are not, as many doctors and vested interests maintain, all in the mind.

Multiple chemical sensitivity (MCS) syndrome, also known as 'environmental illness', has been described as the most puzzling disease of the Eighties (Ann Intern Med, 1988; 322: 675–83). It's also one of the most political because it touches upon the most powerful industries in the world, which have enormous vested interests in keeping the lid on this problem.

Although we have no idea how prevalent the syndrome is, increased sensitivity to a variety of chemicals is thought to be a growing problem (Occup Med, 1987; 2: 663–8; Ann Intern Med, 1988; 322: 675–83). One investigator identified 49 out of 2760 patients, or more than 2 per cent, as suffering from MCS between 1986 and 1991 (Toxicol Ind Health, 1992; 8: 15–9).

What we do know is that many patients with chronic fatigue syndrome/myalgic encephalomyelitis (CFS/ME) or fibromyalgia syndrome (FS) also react to chemicals (Arch Intern Med, 1994; 154: 2049–53); that many of the symptoms of those conditions are similar to those of MCS; and that three-quarters of MCS patients are women (Toxicol Ind Health, 1992; 8: 15–9). High sugar and carbohydrate consumption also appear to make people more susceptible.

Four major groups are most at risk: industrial workers, occupants of crowded buildings, communities with air or water contamination, and people with unique exposure to various chemicals (Ashford NA et al., *Chemical Exposures: Low Levels and High Stakes*, Van Nostrand Reinhold, 1991).

What unites all these diverse people is a collection of bizarre symptoms, affecting many organ systems of the body as soon as someone is exposed to chemicals, including seemingly innocuous ones like perfume. These range from headaches and depression to breathing difficulties, flu-like symptoms, ear, nose and throat disturbances, gastrointestinal problems, musculoskeletal problems like joint pain, and even heart and circulatory disturbances.

The disorder causes a progressive hypersensitivity to a variety of substances. People with MCS cannot tolerate drugs of any variety— prescription or recreational. They react to food, other chemicals and are frequently intolerant of alcohol. In the view of Iris Bell, associate professor in psychiatry, psychology and family community medicine at the University of Arizona, and an expert on MCS, this disorder results from a "time-dependent sensitisation" (TDS), which is somehow triggered and then increases over time.

The principal culprit in MCS is undoubtedly pesticides, especially organophosphates (OPs). Other contaminants include air pollution, such as car exhaust fumes, or carbon monoxide; 'indoor' chemicals such as solvents, found in paints, varnishes, adhesives and cleaning solutions, or fumes from carpets, computers and photocopies, plastics, disinfectants and, of course, tobacco smoke; pesticides and the entire range of substances such as hormones, antibiotics, nitrates and heavy metals that make their way into our food and water supply; and even medical and consumer items like plastics, hairsprays, deodorants and felt-tip pens.

OPs inhibit acetylcholinesterase (AchE), an enzyme that breaks down the neurotransmitter acetylcholine at the junctions between nerve cells. This breakdown apparently precipitates an increased supersensitivity to smell. One medical journal (JNNP, 1993; 56: 943–6) went as far as to suggest that chemical exposure may be behind a number of poorly understood neurological diseases. Pesticides, whether inhaled or ingested, are known to affect the hippocampus, the part of the brain responsible making short-term memory long term.

MCS could also be a general immune reaction to low-dose chemicals caused by a malfunctioning enzyme neural endopeptidase (NEP) in the airways (Toxicol Ind Health, 1992; 8: 221–8). In fact, many MCS patients have nasal problems and inflammation, excessive phlegm and catarrh (Arch Environ Health, 1993; 48: 14–8).

Chemical intoxication also appears to cause porphyrin abnormalities. Porphyria is a metabolic disorder causing excessive excretion of porphyrins, the pigments found in haemoglobin, as well as neurological disturbances and abdominal pain. These neurological symptoms are those usually described by MCS patients, and over 90 per cent of MCS patients have porphyria.

According to the Chemical Injury Information Network, 3750 chemicals can cause this abnormality, as can many antibiotics. Some researchers studying the more powerful generation of antibiotics that tamper with bacterial DNA worry that they could alter the recipient's ability to make porphyrins and also the structure of cells. As one doctor studying the syndrome put it: "If we damage the engine that keeps our cells going, then, of course, we can expect . . . what we see in our [MCS] patients" (Townsend Lett Docs, November 1996).

Another important factor in bringing on MCS could be the interaction between chemicals. Currently, some 70,000 chemicals are in commercial use, with another 1000 or so added every year (Rachel's Environment & Health Weekly, 13 June 1996). New research shows that some combinations of chemicals that disrupt hormone function in animals and humans are far more powerful than any of the chemicals on their own (Science, 1996; 272: 1489–92).

Furthermore, combinations of two or three pesticides turn out to be up to 1600 times as powerful as any individual substance on its own. Chlorodane, which has no ability to disrupt hormone function by itself, has been shown to greatly magnify the hormone-disrupting ability of other chemicals when used in combination. This would affect the 50 or so chemicals used in detergents, plastics and pesticides which have been found to interfere with hormones and normal development, causing changes in sexual preference and behaviour, diminished sperm count or small penises, cancer, and nervous system disorders and birth defects.

The main consequence of slow-motion chemical poisoning is nerve damage (Arch Environ Health, 1994; 9: 37–44; Acta Neurol Scand, 1988; 78 [Suppl]: 1–143; Environ Res, 1993; 60: 124–35). Nervous system disturbances have been found in many MCS patients as a cause of damage to or loss of peripheral vision. Many show electromyographic abnormalities, and develop disturbances in bowel and bladder control (Occup Med State Art Rev, 1987; 2: 669–82). In brain scans, patients exposed to chemicals show changes in brain processes and even in parts of the brain, particularly the frontal and temporal lobes, thalamus and cerebellum (J Toxicol Environ Health, 1994; 41: 275–84). Those exposed to dioxins, solvents or pesticides show a reduced cerebral blood flow (Toxicol Ind Health, 1994; 10: 561–71).

Environmental toxins also cause heart and circulatory problems, including arteriosclerosis, high blood pressure, ischaemic heart disease, heart muscle disease and disturbances of heart muscle rhythm (Occup Med State Art Rev, 1992; 7: 465–78; J Occup Med, 1983; 25: 879–85).

Polyaromatic hydrocarbon levels have also been found to depress lymphocyte function (Toxicol Appl Pharmacol, 1992; 117: 155–64).

A number of prestigious scientists have identified multiple chemical exposure to be behind many of our most puzzling illnesses like CFS/ ME. In 1993, Professor William Rea, author of *Chemical Sensitivity* (Ann Arbor, Michigan: Lewis Publishing), has suggested that reactions to a wide range of chemical substances may lie at the root of ME. Dr Charles Poser, a well-known neurologist from Harvard Medical School, believes that a paradoxical or inappropriate response to medications, one of the main symptoms of MCS, is a very important criterion when making a diagnosis of ME. This suggests that MCS and ME are variations of the same illness (International Conference on CFS, Dublin, 1994).

Or it could be that a high body burden of pesticides is an effect of an illness like CFS/ME. A three-year study in Australia showed a statistically significant connection between the level of organochlorines in the body and the severity of CFS/ME. The high levels of pesticides in the body could be the result of a faulty detoxification system, which results in the CFS/ME (Our Toxic Times, February 1996, as quoted in Townsend Lett Docs).

All in your head

Although orthodox medicine has given the MCS syndrome some legitimacy by identifying it with a label, it still categorises MCS as psychosomatic, that all-purpose rubbish bin into which the medical profession throws all illnesses it doesn't understand. A 1996 report, prepared by a working group from the Royal Colleges of Physicians, Psychiatrists and General Practitioners, claims that as many as three-quarters of the up to one million people believed to suffer from CFS/ME have underlying psychological or psychiatric problems. Food and chemical sensitivities, which may be important triggers in these conditions, are dismissed as 'somatisation disorders'—the conversion of a mental state into a body dysfunction—as though an environmental insult has nothing to do with it.

Psychiatrists have consistently maintained that problems like MCS and other allergic reactions can be explained in terms of psychological or somatisation disorder (BMJ, 1993; 307: 747–8; Clin Exp Allergy, 1995; 25: 503–14). Medical 'authorities' on the subject have even instructed doctors on how to identify and diagnose a variety of disorders in such patients, including the bizarre Munchhausen syndrome by proxy (where the sufferer inflicts fake illnesses on others, say, by adding sugar to a child's urine to produce a diagnosis of diabetes). Nevertheless, many of the studies supposedly proving that MCS is just another term for neurotic are now known to be flawed.

In one study, groups of workers for the aircraft manufacturer

Boeing, based in Seattle, Washington, were found to suffer from psychiatric disorders. Eventually, their problems turned out to be caused by exposure to toxic substances used in manufacturing processes (Am J Psychiatry, 1990; 147: 901–6). This fact has now been acknowledged in a high court judgement in the state of Washington, where the judges decreed that Boeing was not only grossly negligent in the application of phenol resins, but also deliberately disregarded the known facts concerning its health hazards.

In 1994, an analysis of the scientific evidence effectively demolished the notion that MCS is a psychological problem. After reviewing 10 papers published after 1980, which supposedly proved that MCS is all in the head, the analysis identified 15 possible methodological problems; indeed, only one of the 10 studies failed on fewer than eight counts (Arch Environ Health, 1994, 49: 316–25).

Recent studies have now shown that MCS differs from common-or-garden psychiatric complaints in tangible ways. MCS researcher Iris Bell has shown that, unlike classical depression, where symptoms are ongoing, MCS patients experience depression, confusion and general apathy for only minutes or hours at a time, and then only after exposure to chemicals. They also experience clumsiness and balance problems, which don't occur in psychiatric illnesses like depression. Few MCS sufferers have any prior history of mental illness (Our Toxic Times, February 1996, as quoted in Townsend Lett Docs).

A new diagnostic tool has also provided a unique neurological signature for MCS. Brain scans using SPECT (single photon emission computed tomography), which measures blood flow in the brain, have shown that exposure to neurotoxic substances, solvents and pesticides appear to significantly impair cerebral function. In one study, scan patterns from patients exposed to chemicals "differed markedly" from those suffering from depression (Our Toxic Times, February 1996, as quoted in Townsend Lett Docs).

Although the medical establishment has argued that no scientific studies have ever established the existence of MCS, researchers from the state of Washington performed a series of double-blind studies on chemically sensitive patients 34 years ago. In this 1963 study, the reaction of patients to plastic food containers was tested after all chemical irritants had been withdrawn from their food and environment for a week. When the plastic was reintroduced, three of the 14 subjects displayed what we now consider the classical symptoms of MCS.

These studies were repeated until it was proved without a doubt that the patients were reacting to the plastic (Our Toxic Times, March 1996, as quoted in Townsend Lett Docs).

The undefinition of MCS

Patients with MCS don't simply have a doubting medical profession to contend with—they must also put up with pressure brought to bear by an industry with an enormous vested interest in demonstrating that chemicals can't make people ill.

In 1996, a workshop on MCS was held in Berlin, Germany. Although co-sponsored by the World Health Organization, the United Nations Environmental Program (UNEP) and the International Labor Program (ILP), lending the event the appearance of an objective international environmental taskforce, the actual sponsor was the International Program on Chemical Safety (IPCS), an organisation firmly on the side of industry. Most of the workshop attendees represented federal institutions, and the chemical and pharmaceutical industries, such as Bayer AG, BASF, Monsanto and Coca-Cola International (CFIDS Chron, 1996; Spring: 5).

No representatives of chemically injured people were permitted to attend. Several of the 17 'experts' convened by the IPCS testified for chemical companies against the existence of MCS.

The workshop concluded that unexplained environmental intolerances do indeed exist, but recommended that the syndrome be labelled 'idiopathic environmental intolerances'—in other words, that the 'intolerances' are self-origninated or of unknown origin—and, thus, to be treated as psychological problems.

The workshop's proposals were subsequently rejected by a large group of international scientists. The WHO, UNEP and ILP distanced themselves from these conclusions as well (Zeit Umweltmed, 1997; 5: 20–2).

Nevertheless, the 'idiopathic environmental intolerances' label has stuck. In Germany, where a significant number of people suffer from MCS, IEI is now considered synonymous for a wide range of so-called 'ill-defined diseases', including sick building syndrome, clinical ecology syndrome, Gulf War syndrome, CFS/ME and fibromyalgia as well as MCS. In a new environmental journal (Umweltmed Forsch Prax, 1996; 1: 229–38), the author claims that the first port of call for any MCS sufferer should be the psychiatrist's couch.

Toxic chemicals

Nowadays, these chemicals are to us what viruses were a century ago—the hidden enemy and the source of much illness. In our everyday life, we are immersed in chemicals. At the last count, there were 70,000 of them out there.

There is now sick building syndrome, wood preservative syndrome, solvent intolerance, chemically associated immune dysfunction, Gulf War syndrome—not to mention the more obtuse appellations such as ecological disease, clinical ecology syndrome, chronic fatigue syndrome/myalgic encephalomyelitis, fibromyalgia, and, our latest, multiple chemical sensitivity—all hinting at environmental causes.

Yet, despite increasing evidence that chemicals are making many people ill, the medical establishment stubbornly hangs on to microbes as the one and only source of illness, and consider any other problem the stuff of the sufferer's fevered imagination.

This was the conclusion of the 1996 Royal College's report on CFS/ME and MCS problems. Nevertheless, the editor of The Lancet,

Dr Richard Horton, took a brave step forward by arguing: "Somehow I cannot accept that pesticides, sprays and gases are the harmless accoutrements of today's life. But how do we prove it one way or the other?"

Although some good scientific studies have already proved that some people are hypersensitive to chemicals, the crux of the problem really lies in finding out exactly how these chemicals damage us and which of our chemical pathways they disturb.

There is no way to determine, for instance, if a single chemical disrupts hormones, say, simply by examining its molecular makeup. You have to subject it to a battery of tests—which, incidentally, have yet to be devised. Just consider, for a moment, the prospect of testing 70,000 chemicals one by one.

An even more mountainous problem concerns the effect of these substances in tandem. We now know that the combined effect of two or three pesticides at low levels, as might be found in most ordinary modern environments, can magnify by up to 1600 times the effect of any insecticide on its own. So, that means it makes sense to test these chemicals in combination. But, as Rachel's Environment & Health Weekly pointed out (13 June, 1996):

"To test just the commonest 1000 toxic chemicals in unique combinations of three would require at least 166 million different experiments (and this disregards the need to study varying doses). Even if each experiment took just one hour to complete and 100 laboratories worked round the clock, seven days a week, testing all possible unique three-way combinations of 1000 chemicals would still take over 180 years to complete."

That staggering notion requires all of us to shout a little louder at the chemical industry. At the moment, most chemicals are innocent until proven guilty.

Consumers must demand that far fewer chemicals be used—and only those about which the most is known—and that pesticides be employed only for emergencies. It should be expected that the manufacturers must bear the burden of proof to prove that a chemical is safe before it can be circulated.

Perhaps most important, we must no longer allow the deadly triad of the medical, pharmaceutical and chemical giants to pretend that the beginnings of an environmental plague are all in our heads, a pretense that allows them to get away with murder.

Toxins and fat

Toxins have an affinity for fat. They like to lodge themselves in the fat that is contained within the fat cells around the body. As a rule, the body doesn't like to let the concentration of potentially harmful substances rise too high.

One way to reduce toxicity is to clear them more quickly. However, if this is not appropriate or just doesn't work quickly enough, the body's only other option is to 'dilute' the toxins. As the toxins generally sit around in the fat cells, one way for the body to accommodate them is to make the fat cells bigger.

Another way that toxins may be diluted in the body is when fluid accumulates. Fluid retention, or oedema (swollen ankles, puffy hands and face) is a common factor in food intolerance, which is itself a frequent underlying feature in toxicity.

Toxins can also interfere with the body's metabolic reactions, causing them to stall and thus causing weight to accumulate.

Chapter 6
Household cleaners

Most household cleaners are a witch's brew of toxic chemicals, industrial waste and carcinogens when all you need are some old-fashioned cleaning staples and a bit of elbow grease.

For years, the concern over the use of household cleaners has focused on the impact they have on our environment. However, many of the chemicals used in household cleaners—from dish detergent to toilet cleaner and air fresheners—are known to poison people as well as plant life. In addition to harsh detergents, consider the following common ingredients in household cleaners:

◆ **Formaldehyde**, used as a preservative, is a known human carcinogen.

◆ **Naphthalene**, a petroleum distillate, is poisonous to humans and a potential carcinogen.

◆ **Paradichlorobenzene**, sometimes used as a disinfectant, is irritating to the skin, eyes and throat, can cause drowsiness and headache, and may cause liver cancer in some animals.

◆ **Propellants, such as butane, isobutane and propane**, are used in all pressurised sprays and are potent neurotoxins.

◆ **Phenol, also known as carbolic acid**, is corrosive, poisonous, able to cause central nervous system disorders and circulatory changes, and a suspected carcinogen.

◆ **Perfumes derived from petrochemicals** (many of which are designated hazardous waste by government agencies) can cause a variety of symptoms, including mood swings, central nervous system disorders, allergic and asthmatic reactions, headaches and more.

◆ **Colours and dyes**, usually made from coal tar, are carcinogenic, and can also contain impurities such as lead and arsenic, also known to cause cancer.

Most of us would agree that advances in home hygiene have been responsible for better health all round. But few people are aware that household cleaning products are anything but good for human health.

Over the years, scientific attention has focused on the environmental impact of the detergents, solvents and phosphates so commonly found in household products. We know what happens to birds, plants, frogs and the ozone layer when these toxins are released into the air and waterways. But little attention has been paid to the impact on human health.

Emerging evidence is that the cleaners, detergents, polishes and air fresheners can make us sick. Children, the elderly, pregnant women and those whose health is already compromised by allergies and asthma are especially at risk.

The substances found in everyday cleaning products run the gamut from toxic to corrosive to poisonous. Unfortunately, manufacturers are not required to list specific ingredients on the label, so consumers may never know what they're getting.

Any substance that comes into contact with your skin, that you inhale, and that you wash down the drain and into the soil will ultimately end up inside your body. Awareness of this has led to a movement to find better alternatives and to 'clean up' the cleaners we use.

However, in an effort to find alternatives to using detergents to do other jobs like the laundry, a number of gadgets, such as wash balls and washing discs, have flooded the market. These products claim to be safe and effective alternatives to detergent. They ionise the water (which all surfactants do), changing its molecular structure so that dirt is drawn naturally away from the clothes. Many manufacturers suggest that, by using these gadgets, we can throw away those heavy boxes and bottles of harmful detergents, and replace it with a mysterious 'green', economical ball.

In 1999, the US Federal Trade Commission (FTC) published the consumer alert *Wash Daze: Laundry Gadgets Won't Lighten the Load*. In it, they concluded that such products "do little more than clean out your wallet" and that "At best, they are marginally better than washing your clothes in water alone, but certainly not as effective as using laundry detergent. At worst, they are completely useless."

The report pointed out that getting your clothes clean was not about gadgets, but about following care-label instructions and using the right amount of detergent for the job. The FTC didn't comment on the differences among traditional detergents. However, it is generally accepted that those based on vegetable—rather than petrochemical—detergents can clean just as effectively and tend to biodegrade more quickly.

Equally, non-biological detergents, which don't contain enzymes—live bacteria included to tackle protein-based stains like sweat and blood—are generally just as effective as their biological counterparts. Enzymes are a major source of allergic skin and respiratory reactions to laundry powder, and should be avoided by sensitive individuals.

Most of us are used to buying our cleaning products off supermarket shelves. When we think of alternatives, often the first place we look is back in the supermarket—where 'green' alternatives are often pretty thin on the ground.

So why not consider making your own? The simplest (and cheapest) ingredients are often all that is needed for the majority of household cleaning jobs.

If you're the kind of person who just has to have a shiny new bottle for everything, consider the Clean House Clean Planet Kit. This kit contains five new bottles—two spray, two squeezy and one jar-type—each with a recipe on the label to help you make safe cleaning products for glass and mirrors, floors, and the bath and kitchen, as well as natural furniture polish from ingredients like baking soda, club soda, olive oil and vinegar. Also included is a bottle of Dr Bronner's peppermint soap for those mixtures that require a bit of detergent power. The bottles can be refilled again and again, and costs £17.95 from 21st Century Health (020 7935 5440).

Keep your house clean naturally

The best way to keep your home clean is to not let grease and grime build up in the first place. A quick regular wipedown is still the best way to prevent surfaces from getting sticky, greasy and grimy. It will also make doing big jobs, like ovens and hobs, a lot easier in the long run.

To limit your exposure to the chemicals in household cleaners, try the following options:

◆ *Use hot water.* Many people forget that hot water and steam are among the best and most effective household cleaners. In addition, it is usually elbow grease, not the chemicals, that really gets the job done.

◆ *Dilute (and dilute again).* Most liquid detergents and soaps can be made into useful all-purpose cleaners by simply diluting them. To expose yourself to a minimum of chemicals, try using an ecological, vegetable-based dish detergent or, even better, a liquid castile soap, well diluted in water.

◆ *Limit your use of sprays* (even pump sprays of homemade mixtures) to those hard-to-get-at places to reduce the amount of chemicals you inhale.

◆ *For tough grease, make a strong solution containing*:
   $1/2$ tsp washing soda (sodium carbonate, soda ash or salsoda)
   2 tbsp distilled white vinegar
   $1/4$ tsp liquid soap or dish detergent (alternatively, 1 tsp soap flakes)
   2 cups (500 mL) hot water.
Add a few drops of essential oils if you wish. This can be used neat or put into a spray bottle for those hard-to-reach places. Always wear gloves when working with washing soda.

◆ *Make a simple scouring powder from 200 g of bicarbonate of soda*. Keep in an airtight jar. If you like, add 10 drops of an essential oil like lemon, grapefruit, mandarin, tea tree, rose, peppermint or lavender and mix well.

◆ *Make a stain-removing scouring powder with*:
   8 oz bicarbonate of soda
   3 oz borax
   3 tbsp soap flakes (lightly crushed).
This will get rid of all but the most stubborn stains. To increase the bleaching power of this mixture, add 3 tbsp sodium perborate (available at healthfood shops), which is a bleach. You should wear gloves when using this formula to avoid skin irritation.

◆ *Make a stronger cleaner, using a mixture of liquid soap and trisodium phosphate (TSP)*. To 1 $1/2$ pints of warm-to-hot water, add:
   1 tsp liquid soap
   1 tsp TSP
   1 tsp borax
   1 tsp distilled white vinegar.

TSP is effective against grease and mildew, but is also a strong skin irritant, so you should wear protective gloves when using it.

Alternatives for the bathroom

Not even the darkest recesses of your toilet need attacking with so many detergents and disinfectants. And it's not the cleaning products, but the tools you use with them that are important.

The first thing to do is invest in a good-quality toilet bowl brush, one with stiff bristles which can be stored in a unit that allows it to airdry between uses. You can clean your toilet with any detergent and get the job done. Plain, diluted vegetable-based dishwashing liquid or castile soap is ideal, or try the following:

◆ *Make a simple toilet cleaner with*:
   4 oz vegetable-based dishwashing liquid or castile soap
   2 cups baking soda
   2 oz water
   2 tbsp white vinegar.
You can even add $1/2$ tsp of essential oils like peppermint, lemon, pine, tea tree or eucalyptus to give it a fresh clean scent. Mix the ingredients together (adding the vinegar last) and put them into a thoroughly rinsed squeezable bottle. This mixture can be used inside and outside the toilet bowl.

◆ *To remove mineral deposits*, add a cup (250 mL) of white vinegar to the toilet bowl, then toss in a handful of baking soda. Let this bubble away for 10–15 minutes before giving the bowl a good scrub and flush.

◆ *An overnight soak*. A simple way to clean the toilet bowl is to pour half-a-cup of borax straight into the bowl, use your brush to give the bowl a quick once over, then leave it overnight.

◆ *Another overnight soak.* At night, put two effervescent 1000 mg vitamin C tablets (unflavoured), or a mixture of 2 tbsp each of citric acid and bicarbonate of soda, into the toilet bowl. In the morning, brush around the bowl and flush. This helps to remove scum below the waterline.

◆ *Buy washable shower curtains.* Wash them regularly to prevent soap and mildew buildup. When they become really scummy, spray them with undiluted distilled vinegar before washing to get rid of soap residues. If you have a glass shower door, wipe it down after each use with a superabsorbent sponge cloth or, better yet, a squeegee.

◆ *Wipe down tiles and glass doors regularly.* This will prevent soap scum buildup. Sounds like too much work? Actually, it only takes about 30 seconds.

Chapter 7
Pesticides

L evels of pesticides found in our bodies are dangerously above those reckoned to be safe, and may be responsible for many cancers and the epidemic of infertility.

Lately, the British press has sounded warnings about the dangers of excessive pesticide levels in carrots and lettuce. But researcher Tuula Tuormaa, on behalf of Foresight, the Association of Preconceptual Care, has discovered that pesticide dangers lurk in everything we put on the table.

Nowadays, it's estimated that the industry worldwide is producing about 45,000–50,000 different pesticides, based on about 600 active ingredients. In one year alone, 23,504 tonnes of active ingredients were sold by UK pesticide manufacturers, which translates into 420 g of chemicals for every man, woman and child in Britain.

During crop growth, pesticides are used as insecticides, herbicides and fungicides. Most of what we eat is subjected to multiple doses of these chemicals. Cereal crops such as wheat are doused an estimated five to eight times during the growing season; with some vegetables and fruit crops, 10–15 sprays are the norm.

Then, after harvesting, most cereal, fruit and vegetable crops are doused again with several pesticides to protect them from storage diseases. This particular treatment, dubbed the 'bucket-and-shower' method, is a fairly crude affair: the pesticides, mixed with freshly harvested produce, are poured into the storage container with food that has already been treated. So even though the actual harvest may have been relatively uncontaminated with pesticides, the casual way that it is treated in storage can add a considerable amount of pesticide residues to the food by the time it reaches your table.

Pesticides are also used during livestock production either as preventative 'animal medicines', such as sheep-dip, warble-fly dressings and lice treatments, or as veterinary pesticides to control flies and other insects in the livestock houses.

But, of course, pesticides aren't simply used in food. Local authorities use a great variety of different pesticides in their parks, gardens, lawns, golf courses and other recreational areas. Besides railroad contractors, who spray thousands of kilos of pesticides, largely atrazine and simazine, onto railways and their embankments, herbicides and chemicals such as sodium chlorate, dichlorobenzene and diquat are applied around canals and various waterways to remove excessive weeds.

Modern building practices use lindane as an active ingredient in their current wood-preservation treatments. Electric cables are doused with an insecticide called aldrin (a chlorinated naphthalene derivative). Different pesticides are also widely used at all stages of forest management. And these days, most homeowners spread pesticides around their own domestic gardens.

Pesticides are also present in a vast number of different manufactured products, such as wallpaper pastes, wooden furniture, DIY products and natural-fibre textiles. New carpets are often treated with mothproofing chemicals, including common insecticides such as pyrethrums and lindane. Pesticides even seem to be present in our bathroom cabinets and medicine chests—warfarin, widely used for the prevention of blood clots, originally was a rodenticide.

Organochlorides (OC) are one of the earliest of the mass-produced pesticides, and include DDT (dichlorodiphenyltrichloroethane), lindane, dieldrin and aldrin. OCs are particularly harmful because they tend to collect in fatty tissue and don't readily break down. Because they are so tenacious, this group of pesticides is able to accumulate along the food chain, from insects to birds, to fish and, finally, to larger mammals, including humans (MAFF, *Report of the Working Party on Pesticide Residues*, London: HMSO, 1989). Because of this cumulative danger, the use of OCs was eventually banned in the US in 1971. In the UK, they were subject to a voluntary ban from 1974 to 1978, after which they were finally removed by law. Even though they are no longer used, since the 1980s, the levels of OCs in food have remained fairly stable, mainly because they are still used in industry or used illegally in farming.

In 1979, a study which analysed foods found high levels of dieldrin in milk and potato, as well as lindane in meat, milk and poultry. Some of the samples exceeded the current EC recommended maximum residue level (MRL) (WPRR, *Report of the Working Party on Pesticide Residues*, London, 1988–1989).

Furthermore, OC residues such as DDT have been found in the fat tissue of all people tested. In 1977, the average DDT contamination in men was 2.6 ppm (parts per million) and 1.6 ppm in women, both levels exceeding the current official EC MRL. In some men, DDT levels were 15 times over the EC legal limit, and some women had levels that were 17 times in excess (MAFF, *Report of the Working Party on Pesticide Residues (1977–81)*, London: HMSO, 1982). More worrying, traces of lindane and dieldrin were detected in a 1979–1980 UK survey of human milk samples.

Even some infant foods have been found to be contaminated with pesticides. A 1987 Ministry of Agriculture, Fisheries and Food (MAFF) survey of 50 infant foods detected that 18 out of 31 samples of infant rusks contained pirimiphos methyl, and three samples of cow's milk contained dieldrin at levels exceeding the EC MRL. These findings are particularly alarming because they show that exposure to pesticides can commence at the very beginning of your life, when you are most vulnerable to the effects of these poisons.

New evidence also suggests that OCs, which seem to have mild oestrogenic properties, can even bring on labour. Studies in Brazil and in India have shown that levels of DDT are significantly higher both in miscarried fetuses and in premature babies compared with those born full-term (Acta Paediatr Scand, 1981; 700: 925–8).

All of us are exposed to excessive levels of pesticides because the levels in our food and water are poorly controlled. The 1985–1988 report of the MAFF Working Party on Pesticide Residues on animal products found that the most commonly detected pesticide residues in animal meat were pp'DDE, a metabolite of DDT, and gamma-HCH, a form of hexachlorocyclohexane. Because these residues were most commonly found in lamb, it's likely that they get into the food chain through the use of DDT and HCH in sheep-dip.

The same survey in 1982–1986 on vegetables and fruit found that 37 out of 67 samples of potatoes analysed contained residues of tecnazene in excess of the EC's recommended MRL. Tecnazene is widely used for the prevention of various storage diseases. In fact, pure bran, because it is positioned outside the grain, has been found to be contaminated with pesticides at levels that are three to four times higher than that of the whole grain. The same was found with apple and pear crops, of which approximately 80 per cent are held in long-term storage before distribution.

A survey conducted by the Association of Public Analysts in 1983 found that one-third of all fruit and vegetables sampled were contaminated with pesticide residues (*The BMA Guide to Pesticides, Chemicals and Health*, London: Edward Arnold Publishers, 1992).

A recent survey conducted on drinking-water quality identified 298 water supplies in the UK that were contaminated with pesticides, with nearly a quarter exceeding the maximum admissible concentration (MAC) of pesticide residues. Sixteen different active pesticide ingredients were detected.

Besides pesticides and other industrial pollutants, nitrates are also widely detected in drinking water supplies. This is due to the ever-increasing amounts of nitrogen-based fertilisers being added to the soil. In the late 1930s, 60,000 tonnes of nitrogen fertilisers were spread on agricultural land in the UK each year. By 1985, this had increased 250 times to 1,580,000 tonnes (Town Country Plan, 1987; 56: 131–2). Because only about half of the fertilisers applied are taken up by the crop, the other half is lost into the atmosphere, or leaches into surface or ground water reservoirs (Assoc Quart Rev, September 16–18, 1985). Presently, it's estimated that approximately one million people in the UK are exposed to nitrate levels in drinking water that exceed the present MAC level, which may quadruple by the turn of the century.

Considering how pervasive pesticide use is these days, what is this long-term exposure doing to you? The London Food Commission conducted a thorough toxicological survey of the active ingredients currently permitted for use by UK pesticide manufacturers. Almost 40 per cent of pesticides currently in use were linked with at least one adverse effect. Out of 426 chemicals listed, 68 were found to be carcinogenic, 61 are capable of mutating genes, 35 have various reproductive effects, ranging from impotence to a variety of birth defects, and 93 can cause skin irritation and similar, milder complications. The most frequently used and troublesome pesticides are herbicides, especially the carboxyacid and phenylurea groups, as well as chlorinated solvents.

Numerous studies show a higher incidence of cancers and related disorders in individuals who are occupationally exposed to pesticides (J Cancer Inst, 1981; 66: 461–4). These include cancers of the lung (J Toxicol Environ Health, 1981; 8: 1027–40), kidney and testicle (Scand J Work Environ Health, 1986; 12: 630–1), leukaemias and multiple types of tumours (Am J Epidemiol, 1971; 94: 307–10), non-Hodgkin's and malignant lymphomas (Lancet, 1981; ii: 579), soft-tissue sarcomas (Br J Cancer, 1979; 39: 711–7) and brain tumours (J Occup Med, 1982; 26: 906–8).

Beside occupational exposure, pesticides seem able to cause cancer if you are chronically exposed from babyhood (Natural Resources Defence Council, *Intolerance Risk: Pesticides in our Children's Food*, Washington, DC: NRDC, 1989). Equally worrying are the effects of pesticides on your fertility. The London Food Commission has listed 35 different pesticides that have been linked to adverse reproductive effects in animal studies, including such widely used formulations as aldrin, benomyl, captan, carbaryl, dieldrin, dinoseb, ioxynil, lindane, maneb and paraquat (The London Food Commission, *Food Adulteration and How to Beat it*, Unwin Paperbacks, 1988).

A number of studies suggest that chronic exposure to pesticides can cause damage to the genetic material of your children. This problem became particularly noticeable when it was found that babies born to the US servicemen exposed during the Vietnam war to a defoliant called Agent Orange (2,4,5-T, mixed with dieldrin) were found to have an extremely high overall rate of birth defects, including spina bifida and facial clefts. The partners of these men also had a high rate of miscarriages and stillbirths (Nature, 1983; 302: 208–9). Besides cleft lip and/or palate, the babies suffered from hydrocephaly (accumulation of cerebrospinal fluid in the brain, leading to extreme swelling of the head, brain damage and convulsions) (Ann Esp Pediatr, 1979; 12: 529–33), and various congenital long bone and limb defects (Commun Health Studies, 1986; 10: 1–11).

Organophosphates have also been shown to cause brain degeneration. This includes a number of the 'sclerosing' diseases, such as multiple sclerosis, muscular dystrophy, Wernicke's encephalopathy and Guillain–Barré-like syndromes (J Nutr Med, 1994; 4: 43–82).

Chronic postnatal exposure to organophosphates has been linked with long-term, measurable changes in brain function (Neurotoxicology, 1980; 1: 667–89), aggression, memory difficulties, depression, emotional instability and schizophrenic reactions (Lancet, 1961; *i*: 1371–4).

We also now know that chronic exposure to organophosphates is able to disrupt regulation of our immune systems (J Nutr Med, 1994; 4: 43–82). This may be one reason that chronic exposure has been linked to the development of allergies and other immunoregulatory disorders, such as chronic fatigue syndrome/myalgic encephalomyelitis (CFS/ME) (Behan, data presented at the First International Research Conference on Chronic Fatigue Syndrome, held in Albany, New York in 1992).

The *N*-nitroso pesticides is considered to be among the most powerful chemical carcinogens; they've been found to cause cancer in 39 animal species studied, including primates (Nutr Health, 1983; 2: 1). High nitrite, derived from high nitrate, has been linked with the 'blue baby' syndrome (due to a lack of haemoglobin and, hence, oxygen).

The use of nitrogen-based fertilisers also affects the nutritional value of crops. With the help of such fertilisers, farmers are able to grow an abundance of green foliage that is virtually devoid of essential trace elements (Pfeiffer CC, *Mental and Elemental Nutrients*, New Canaan, CT: Keats Publishing, 1975).

Recent crop and soil investigations found particularly low levels of manganese, zinc and iron in the samples studied (Nutr Health, 1992; 8: 1–16). Manganese deficiency has been linked with congenital malformations (Am J Clin Nutr, 1985; 41: 1042–4), and zinc deficiency can lead to premature delivery and small-for-gestational-age babies (J Orthomolec Med, 1994; 9: 225–43).

Currently, scientists have sacrificed a great number of animals in the cause of attempting to figure out what constitutes a lethal dose of pesticides. However, these animal tests can tell us nothing. Unlike study animals, which are exposed to high levels over the short term, we are exposed intermittently to multiple combinations of pesticide residues over many years at very low doses. Furthermore, humans do not necessarily respond to substances in the same way as animals do. For example, 2-naphthylamine has been found to be a bladder carcinogen in humans and dogs, but not in mice, rats, guinea pigs and rabbits (Matsumura F, *Toxicology of Pesticides*, New York: Plenum Publishing, 1975).

Despite what is supposed to be a scientific advance, pesticides may have only made the insect problem worse. At least 50 different species of weeds are resistant to herbicides, while the number of insecticide-resistant insects are also growing at an alarming rate (Phytoparasitica, 1988; 16: 364; Pest Sci, 1989; 26: 333–58).

Furthermore, pesticides seem to be unnecessary. The US National

Academy of Sciences monitored 14 successful organic farms over five years. Some of the farms, which had not used agrochemicals for 15 years, had corn yields that were 32 per cent higher, and soya bean yields that were 40 per cent higher, than local farms using pesticides (Nat Acad Sci, *Alternative Agriculture*, Washington, DC: NAS, 1989). Another study found that cutting herbicides by 87 per cent did nothing to reduce yields of either wheat or barley (Farmers Weekly, 6 April 1990).

Called-for controls

The World Resources Institute, a Washington-based pressure group, wants stronger government surveillance and controls over the use and marketing of pesticides, particularly when they are used in developing countries. Pesticides should also be tested for their immunotoxicity.

Its new report, 'Pesticides and the Immune System: the Public Health Risks', draws on new data on pesticide use around the world, and its effects on humans and wildlife.

One piece of research, from Moldova, Russia, discovered that farms in the region were using 20 times the world average for pesticides. More than 80 per cent of children there who were known to have been exposed to the pesticides had "significant deviations in more than five immunological parameters". The children were also three times more likely to have infectous diseases of the gastrointestinal tract, and two to fives times more likely suffer some infectious disease. In adults, "the incidence of respiratory, reproductive, and sensory organ diseases was higher than in residents of areas where pesticide use was less".

Reducing your exposure to pesticides

◆ *Eat organic food, including meat, whenever possible*, especially if you are pregnant or conceiving. Organic crops usually contain no pesticide residues.

◆ *Purchase fruits and vegetables from reputable supermarket chains* if you can't afford or don't have access to organic foods. Because chains have strict monitoring and quality control with their farm-produce suppliers, their shelves generally contain food with lower levels of pesticide residues.

◆ *Wash all fruits and vegetables*, especially leafy vegetables and fruits with skins that are eaten. Since washing removes only a small amount of pesticides, peeling is safer. However, even peeling won't remove all residues since some will find their way into the flesh of most fruits and vegetables.

◆ *Always filter your drinking water,* using a good-quality water filter. Even better, drink bottled water that is produced by a reputable manufacturer.

◆ *Look for alternative forms of pest control* for your own use, such as in your garden. A number of firms now produce organic pesticides with no chemicals. Use pesticides only when you are convinced they are absolutely necessary and then apply only enough chemical to do the job.

◆ *Carefully follow any instructions on the labels of pesticides you use.* Store and apply all household and garden chemicals away from food, children and pets.

◆ *Write to your MP today demanding better pesticide-safety controls* (as this issue is currently under debate). Also, demand that food labelling includes the chemicals used to produce the food.

◆ *Vote with your wallet.* Insist on buying only pesticide-free foods. If enough people shout loudly, retailers will listen.

Chapter 8
Microwave ovens

Simon Best, What Doctors Don't Tell You's resident expert on all things electromagnetic, has produced a chilling testimonial to the dangers of microwave ovens. One of the most comprehensive pieces of journalism on this technology, the following chapter makes for grim reading.

Solid scientific evidence suggests that heating food by microwave denatures food of most vital nutrients. Eating food that has been cooked in this manner produces changes in your blood, cells and immune system suggestive of conditions like cancer.

Food that is microwaved tastes so disgusting that manufacturers have to throw in additives, colourings, artificial flavours and other assorted junk to try to approximate the real thing, or attach them onto the packaging, causing the chemicals to melt into the food. It should come as no surprise to anyone that particles of nifty little timesavers, like those plastic cook-in-the-bag containers, end up in popcorn or breakfast cereal when they are heated to this degree.

But if this technology is so dangerous, why haven't we heard anything about it before? The answer is that a few people have been trying to shout loudly about this, but their information has largely been suppressed by supposedly enlightened Western societies like Switzerland.

This is a story not simply about the dangers of a technology universally sold to a public before its effects were studied or comprehended. It is a classic illustration of commercial interests working in collusion with a government and judiciary to place profits before public interest.

The case of Swiss food scientist Dr Hans-Urich Hertel is another shameful chapter in the history of Switzerland. For 10 years, the Swiss have successfully stifled Dr Hertel's voice through a draconian law that prohibits any criticism whatsoever of business that might harm trade. Although this law is supposed to pertain only to statements that are "untrue or misleading", this depends upon who is called upon to make that determination.

What the Swiss law amounts to is a deliberate stifling of free speech and a suppression of any evidence that might potentially put a dent in the turnover of any particular company or industry.

Most disturbing is that the Swiss hold their commercial liberty more sacred than any other. Although the European Court—the court that is supposed to prevail in Europe over those of any individual EU country—has ruled in favour of Hertel, the Swiss court is taking its time about deciding if it intends to take any notice.

Far be it from us to applaud communism, but the irony of this saga is that a repressive and totalitarian regime like Russia in the 1970s was the only one that saw fit to ban a technology that its scientists determined was undeniably dangerous.

Lest we think this can't happen in Britain, a law is about to be passed here which will prohibit criticism of a product unless it can be backed up by scientific evidence. This sounds fine until you consider how research like Hertel's might be received. Some professor with impressive-sounding credentials would probably be wheeled out in court to say that his evidence was not conclusive, and Hertel's voice would be silenced here as well.

Sometimes the laws that are meant to protect us are the very ones that we should most resist. This new law, which is supposed to help deliver the truth about new products and prohibit companies from making false claims, is really about protecting commerce from scientific enquiry. Only time will tell how many British Hertels get muzzled here as well.

Ten-year-old evidence, suppressed by the Swiss courts, shows that food from a microwave can cause worrying changes in the blood.

More recent studies add to the mounting evidence that microwave ovens pose a hazard to your health.

In 1989, Dr Hertel made some worrying discoveries about microwave ovens. Nevertheless, for more than a decade, he has been fighting for the right to let the world know what he has found. The point that he has been desperately trying to make public is vital to consumer interests: Any food eaten that has been cooked or defrosted in a microwave oven can cause changes in the blood indicative of a developing pathological process that is also found in cancer.

Nevertheless, for all this time, Hertel has been effectively gagged by the manufacturers of microwave ovens who have effectively used trade laws and the Swiss court to muzzle him, and have even threatened him with personal ruin. In March 1993, the Canton of Bern Commercial Court, following a complaint filed by the Swiss Association of Dealers for Electroapparatuses for Households and Industry, prohibited Dr Hertel from publicly declaring or writing that microwave ovens were dangerous to health. Flouting the order could incur a fine of up to SF5000 or land him up to a year in prison.

The Swiss Federal Court in Lausanne confirmed the verdict in 1994. The court based its verdict on the Swiss Law Against Unfair Competition, which prohibits "discriminating, untrue, misleading and unnecessarily harming statements against a supplier or his products" (J Nat Sci, 1998; 1: 2–7), a law that solely considers the inhibition of trade *per se* and not malicious intent.

That law effectively muzzles the Swiss press as well, as any statements which could be viewed as critical of microwave ovens could easily lead to litigation. The view of the Swiss on Dr Hertel's findings are not shared by the rest of Europe. In August 1998, the European Court of Human Rights ruled that the gag order issued by the Swiss courts against Dr Hertel was contrary to the right of freedom of expression. The European court also ordered Switzerland to pay a compensation of SF40,000. Despite his victory, which is two years old, Dr Hertel is still waiting for the Swiss courts to reverse their earlier decision and lift a SF8000 fine against him. In the meantime, his explosive discoveries are being corroborated by evidence cropping up here and there all over the world.

Hertel's research

Eleven years ago, Dr Hertel, who had worked for several years for one of the international Swiss food companies, joined forces with Professor Bernard Blanc, of the Federal Institute of Technology, to conduct an extensive research programme into the effects of micro-waved food on humans. Although the programme was turned down by the Swiss National Fund, the two scientists decided to fund a smaller research programme themselves.

They selected eight people from the Macrobiotic Institute at Kientel in Switzerland, all of whom, including Hertel himself, were adherents to strict macrobiotic diets to minimise the presence of confounding elements that could affect blood measures. Except for Hertel, who was 64 at the time, all were aged between 20 and 40. As Hertel told **WDDTY**: "We all lived in the same hotel for eight weeks and there was no smoking, no alcohol and no sex."

At intervals of two to five days, the volunteers received one of eight possible food sources on an empty stomach: raw milk from a biofarm; the same milk conventionally cooked; the same raw milk cooked in a microwave oven; pasteurised milk from conventional sources; raw vegetables from an organic farm; the same vegetables cooked conventionally; the same vegetables frozen and defrosted in a micro-wave; and the same vegetables cooked in a microwave.

Blood samples were taken from each volunteer immediately before eating and then at specified intervals after eating the above preparations.

Significant changes were observed in the blood of those who had consumed microwaved food, including a reduction in all haemoglobin and cholesterol values, both the high-density lipoproteins ('good'

HDL cholesterol) and low-density lipoproteins ('bad' LDL cholesterol) (Nexus, 1995; April/May: 25–7).

There was a more noticeable short-term decrease in lymphocytes (immune system cells) after the ingestion of microwaved food than after the intake of the other foods. In addition, Hertel discovered a strongly significant association between the amount of microwave energy in the test foods and the brightness of certain bacteria which light up (when looked at under a special light) on exposure to the blood from those who'd eaten the food. Hertel concluded that such energy may be passed on to those eating microwaved food.

Besides these effects of microwave heating of food, Hertel also noted non-thermal effects which, he claims, alter cell membrane permeability by changing the electrical potentials between the outer and inner sides of the cell. The damaged cells then become easy prey to viruses, fungi and other microorganisms.

The natural repair mechanisms of cells are also disturbed, which eventually forces the cells to respond to a 'state of emergency' energy supply by switching from aerobic (oxygen-based) to anaerobic (no oxygen) respiration. Thus, instead of producing water and carbon dioxide, the cells then produce hydrogen peroxide and carbon monoxide. In such a situation, Hertel asserts, cells revert from 'healthy oxidation' to an unhealthy 'fermentation' process of energy generation.

Hertel goes on to state that, when food is microwaved, the oven exerts a power input of about 1000 watts or more. The resulting destruction and deformation of the food molecules produces new compounds, called 'radiolytic' compounds, that are unknown in nature. The current received wisdom in scientific circles is that microwaved and other irradiated food does not contain significantly higher levels of radiolytic compounds than that cooked conventionally, but Hertel's results suggest the contrary.

Blood analyses from the study participants also confirmed that all was not well in those eating microwaved food. Samples taken at 7.45 each morning, at 15 minutes after food intake and two hours later showed that erythrocyte (red blood cell), haemoglobin (oxygen-carrying pigment in red blood cells), haematocrit (red cell volume percentage) and leucocyte (white blood cell) measures were all at the lower limits of normal in those eating the microwaved food.

These results are akin to those of individuals with a tendency towards anaemia; the results were more pronounced and statistically significant in the second month of the study. Furthermore, as these values decreased, blood cholesterol levels correspondingly increased.

It's not hard to see why the publication of such results in 1992 might have produced a furore in Switzerland. Nevertheless, the reaction of the Swiss authorities and industry which took him to court and convicted him under their Unfair Competition law remains a shameful chapter in Swiss history. Such was the pressure on Professor Blanc that he felt forced to publicly dissociate himself from the data interpretation given in their joint report shortly after publication. Privately, he admitted to Dr Hertel that he feared for the safety of his family (J Nat Sci, 1998; 1: 2–7).

Despite attempts to shut him up publicly, Dr Hertel's research is available to the public outside of Switzerland through the post or his website (copies available from The World Foundation for Natural Science, Box 632, CH-3000, Bern, Switzerland, tel: +33 438 1158; fax: +33 437 4816; website: www.wffns.org).

Russians ban microwave ovens

After World War II, the Russians also experimented with microwave ovens. From 1957 up to recently, their research was carried out mainly at the Institute of Radio Technology at Klinsk, Byelorussia.

According to US researcher William Kopp, who gathered together much of the results of Russian and German research into this subject, and was apparently persecuted for doing so (J Nat Sci, 1998; 1: 42–3), the following effects were observed by Russian forensic teams:

- Heating prepared meats in a microwave sufficiently for human consumption created:
  - D-nitrosodiethanolamine (a well-known cancer-causing agent)
  - destabilisation of active protein biomolecular compounds
  - a binding effect with radioactivity in the atmosphere.

- Creation of cancer-causing agents within protein hydrolysate compounds in milk and cereal grains.

- Microwave emissions caused alterations in the catabolic (break-down) behaviour of glucoside and galactoside elements within frozen fruits when thawed in a microwave.

- Microwaves altered catabolic behaviour of plant alkaloids when raw, cooked or frozen vegetables were exposed for even very short periods.

- Cancer-causing free radicals were formed within the molecular structures of certain trace minerals in plant substances, especially in raw root vegetables.

- Ingestion of microwaved foods caused a higher percentage of cancerous cells in blood.

- Due to chemical alterations within food substances, malfunctions occurred in the lymphatic system, causing degeneration of the immune system's capacity to protect itself against cancerous growth.

- The unstable breakdown of microwaved foods altered their elemental food substances, leading to disorders in the digestive system.

◆ Those ingesting microwaved foods showed a statistically higher incidence of stomach and intestinal cancers as well as a general degeneration of peripheral cellular tissues, with a gradual break-down of digestive and excretory system function.

Microwave exposure caused significant decreases in the nutritional value of all of the foods studied, particularly:

◆ A decrease in the bioavailability of B-complex vitamins, vitamin C, vitamin E, essential minerals and lipotrophics.

◆ Destruction of the nutritional value of nucleoproteins in meats.

◆ Reduced metabolic activity of alkaloids, glucosides, galactosides and nitrilosides (all basic plant substances in fruits and vegetables).

◆ Marked acceleration of the structural disintegration in all foods (Perceptions, 1996; May/June: 30–3).

As a result, microwave ovens were banned in Russia in 1976, although the ban was lifted after *Perestroika*.

Recent research

While some of the above findings remain to be replicated, other research in Britain and the US has unearthed other possible hazards. In 1990 at the University of Leeds, two scientists in the Department of Medical Microbiology studied the uneven heating that can be caused by microwave ovens. They found that the salt content in a specified portion of mashed potatoes influenced its inside temperature—the greater the salt content, the lower the temperature.

The authors concluded that "the poor penetration of microwaves into the test food with high ionic concentrations may result from the induction of electrical/ionic flow in the surface of the food. This would also explain why commercial food heated in microwaves commonly boils on the surface but is cool on the inside" (Nature, 1990; 344: 496).

A case was reported in 1991 of a hospitalised patient in Tulsa, Oklahoma, who died of anaphylaxis (an immediate generalised hypersensitivity 'allergic'-type shock) after receiving a transfusion of blood which had been warmed in a microwave oven. The irradiation appears to have altered the blood in some way and caused the patient's death (J Nat Sci, 1998; 1: 2–7).

In August 1989, British government research showed that *Listeria* and other potentially fatal bacteria can survive in microwave-cooked food, even if instructions are followed (Food Bus, 1989; 20: 12).

Other US research has shown that the practice of reheating leftover food in a microwave is potentially dangerous. Researchers investigating an outbreak of *Salmonella* among those attending a picnic in 1992 discovered that, of 30 people who took home leftover meat, all 10 who used a microwave became ill. None of a further 10 persons who used a conventional oven or skillet to reheat the pork became ill.

The researchers concluded that, compared with conventional methods of reheating food, microwave ovens offered no preventative protection from illness (Am J Epidemiol, 1994; 139: 903–9).

Not all evidence has been negative. Scientists at a nutrition and food research institute in Zeist, The Netherlands, carried out a 13-week study into the effects of microwaved food on the blood chemistry and other health indicators in rats, and apparently found no adverse effects (Food Chem Toxicol, 1995; 33: 245–56). Nevertheless, such animal studies may not necessarily apply to human health.

Beware of leaking additives

Another problem with microwaved food is that it is low in colour and flavour compared with conventionally cooked food, especially in foods containing pastry. This has encouraged the development of microwavable food additives to artificially produce the colours and flavours consumers have come to expect.

As Australian academics John Ashton and Ron Laura state in their strongly recommended book *The Perils of Progress* (Zed Books, London, 1999): "An example of one new type of flavour-producing technology designed for use in microwave ovens is susceptors. These devices are usually glued to the packaging of microwavable foods and are used to achieve local areas of high temperature. This has the effect of browning the food during microwave cooking. A subtle side-effect of some of the pre-1992 susceptor devices involved the release of small amounts of a toxic chemical, bisphenol-A-diglycidyl ether (BADGE), into the food during microwaving. BADGE was a component of the cold cure adhesive used to fix susceptors to packaging."

The authors cite a 1992 study of 52 samples of pizza in which nine samples of susceptors used in one brand contained BADGE at concentrations between 0.2–0.3 per cent. The chemical was found to migrate into the pizza when they were cooked in their packaging according to the instructions (Food Add Contam, 1995; 12: 779–87).

Other research has shown that a large number of chemicals are released from susceptors packed together with foods such as pizzas, waffles and French fries intended for a microwave. One study identified 44 different volatile chemicals, including the carcinogen benzene (AOAC Int, 1993; 76: 1268–75). Another toxic chemical observed to migrate from packaging into food when microwaved is benzophenone, a component of the ink on the printed paperboard (Food Add Contam, 1994; 11: 231–40).

Bread and breakfast cereals are often sold in waxed bags for easy heating in a microwave. However, a recent study showed that following the instructions on the packaging resulted in 60 per cent of the wax being transferred to the food (Food Add Contam, 1994; 11: 79–89).

The PVC (polyvinyl chloride) plastic films that cover food during microwave cooking have been found to release plasticisers into the food to such a degree that a 1996 study recommended that PVC should not be used in direct contact with food during cooking (Badeka AB, Kontominas MG, 1996, as cited in Ashton J, Laura RS, *The Perils of Progress* London: Zed Books, 1999: 68).

The message seems clear. Don't cook food in a microwave oven, especially for children, unless there is a genuine need for urgency. Resist the slick and misleading advertising offering the 'quick fix' for your 'busy life'. Realise that the body requires wholesome food prepared in as wholesome a way as possible to function optimally. To the degree that you consume less-than-wholesome food, your body organs and processes will be adversely affected, leading to degeneration and disease. Treat your body like a Rolls-Royce, not a waste-disposal bin.

Where do microwaves come from?

Some believe that microwave ovens were developed during World War II by the Germans to enable easy food production in their submarines; others say that the same scientists developed these devices to support mobile operations during their invasion of the Soviet Union. Whatever the case, the invention dates from WWII.

After the War, the technology was taken back to the US and developed, resulting in the first domestic oven launched onto the American market in 1952 by the Raytheon company. Since then, the technology has been promoted all over the world with virtually no research by the relevant authorities in any country into its possible harmful effects.

It was not until the 1970s that the first reports started appearing, casting doubt on the safety of food cooked in a microwave. Microscopy studies using microwaved broccoli and carrots revealed that the molecular structures of nutrients were deformed to the point of destroying cell walls whereas, in conventional cooking, cell structures remain intact (J Food Sci, 1975; 40: 1025–9).

How a microwave works

A microwave oven uses a device called a magnetron tube, which causes an electron beam to oscillate at very high frequencies, thus producing microwave radiation. Domestic and commercial units use a frequency of 2.45 gigahertz (GHz) with an output of 400–900 watts for a typical domestic oven, which has a power supply designed to deliver 4000-volt pulses to the magnetron. The 2.45-GHz frequency is used because water absorbs electromagnetic energy quickest and at maximum at this frequency, thus allowing food containing water to be heated up quickly.

The molecules within the food are forced to align themselves with the rapidly alternating field and to oscillate around their axis. Heat is produced from the considerable intermolecular friction. Microwaves are beamed from the magnetron into the oven compartment, where they heat the food from the inside out—unlike conventional ovens, which do the reverse. Heating from the inside first can give rise to cold spots, hence the need to rotate the dish constantly.

The maximum leakage level allowed under current standards is a power density of 5 milliwatts per square centimetre at a distance of 5 cm from the oven door. This limit is based on standards for microwave radiation and is disputed by those who argue that non-thermal effects of microwave radiation should be taken into account when tallying radiation levels (as, for example, with mobile phones). The door of the microwave oven itself should be checked periodically to ensure that it is not leaking excessively.

Protect yourself against radiation

If you must continue to use a microwave oven:

◆ Have it checked regularly for leakage, especially the door, which is prone to do so.

- Never open the door while the oven is on.

- Stand at least three feet away (especially children) from the oven when in use to avoid the cumulative effects of even low-level exposure. The lens of the eye is most at risk from prolonged microwave exposure because it has no way of dissipating the energy thermally or otherwise.

- Avoid microwave cooking of frozen foods and commercially prepared meals, especially if they are to be cooked in their packaging.

- Use non-PVC cooking containers whenever possible.

- Discourage growing children from eating microwaved food or using a microwave.

- Be aware that the majority of restaurant food is now microwaved using large commercial ovens. These pose even greater potential risks to users, and those who use them should be warned.

Chapter 9
Mobile phones

Mobile phones are safe or, at least, that's what the industry would like you to believe. However, a number of new research projects around the world are coming up with disturbing results—including every possibility from brain damage to asthma. These studies are so worrying that an expert group, headed by Dr Alastair McKinlay of the UK's National Radiological Protection Board (NRPB), has concluded that a £20 million, five-year research programme is warranted.

Drs Henry Lai and Narendra Singh at Washington State University observed that exposure of the brain cells of rats to low-level microwaves (such as those found in microwave ovens and mobile phones) produced single- and double-strand breaks in DNA. With both pulsed-wave and continuous-wave radiation, they found an increase in both types of DNA strand breaks after only four hours of exposure (Int J Radiat Biol, 1996; 69: 513–21).

In humans, cumulative DNA damage in cells has been associated with cancer, Alzheimer's disease, Huntington's disease and Parkinson's disease. In Australia, Dr Peter French, one of Australia's top cell biologists and director of the Centre for Immunology at St Vincent's Hospital in Sydney, has found a dramatic reduction in brain proteins after irradiation of certain brain cells at mobile-phone frequencies. After irradiating laboratory culture dishes of brain cells, using antennae that gave off frequencies similar to that of a mobile phone for 10 minutes a day for a week, certain skeletal bone proteins were reduced by as much as 70 per cent.

Most significantly, the researchers report that, when the damaged cells were subsequently cultured, the damage was never repaired—not even after many cell generations.

Extending his research to lung function, Dr French has observed the effects of irradiation of mast cells in the test tube. These are the cells which deal with inflammatory responses. Under attack from an antigen such as dust or pollen, these cells produce histamine, which constricts the bronchial tube and can trigger an attack of asthma.

French also found that when mast cells were irradiated at mobile phone frequencies for 10 minutes over seven days, they were so irreversibly damaged that exposure to an antigen would produce double the level of histamine than normal.

There have also been many complaints lodged by users. In the UK, at least 100 British Telecom engineers have called up an information service after being issued with mobiles to report headaches, poor short-term memory and concentration, tingling, burning or twitching of the skin on the side of their face nearest the phone, eye problems including 'dry eye', causing irritation on blinking and buzzing in their ears. These symptoms occurred not only while actually using the phone, but also on waking up during the night.

Mobile phone manufacturers are increasingly replacing the original analogue (continuous-wave) phone with the digital (pulsed-wave) variety—mainly for performance and security reasons. Both operate at between 800–900 megahertz (MHz), but the digital ones emit a series of pulses. Research has shown that pulsed microwaves are far more biologically active and penetrative than continuous-wave radiation of the same frequency and power level. Certain digital phones (Global System Mobile GSM and Personal Communications Network PCN) can operate at twice that frequency.

The current UK guidance on the safety of mobile phones by the NRPB is based on the specific absorption rate (SAR), which is based on the heating-up effect of this radiation, and aimed at preventing a rise in temperature of more than 2–4 watts per kilogram (kg) of body weight. However, 'hot spots' of increased absorption can occur in various parts of the body, notably the head, depending on how the phone is held and the size of the head.

Although the NRPB states a safe level of 10 watts/kg for any 10 g of head tissue for both industry workers and the general public, this level is five times higher than the standard adopted by the rest of Europe's CENELEC (European Committee for Electrotechnical Standardization). Digital cellular phones can emit considerably more than 2 watts/kg (CENELEC's upper limit) into head tissue during their output pulses, but they are still deemed to comply because of the way that the power pulses are averaged.

Dr John Dennis, former assistant director of the NRPB, has admitted that the maximum power transmitted by mobile phones may need to be reduced for those with smaller heads.

The shields

Research is not concentrating solely on the hazards of electromagnetic radiation (EMR), but also on how to reduce or prevent exposure. French scientists have presented evidence to show how a new type of antenna protected chick embryos from mobile phone radiation.

Dr Madeleine Bastide and her colleagues at Montpellier University exposed chicken embryos to radiation from a mobile phone, measuring the ELF (0–300 Hz) and VLF (300 Hz–30 MHz) range. They observed that the exposed group suffered a 72 per cent higher death rate than the unexposed group (12 per cent). The distribution of the dead embryos was essentially around the source of the phone radiation. (The same researchers have reported depressed immune system function in chickens from VDU radiation.)

In the second stage of this experiment, chick embryos were again exposed to similar radiation except that, for one group, the phone was fitted with a Tecno AO antenna (made by the French company Tecnosphere). The embryo death rate for the protected group was 29 per cent *vs* 57 per cent in the unprotected group, indicating that the antenna had successfully shielded the embryos. Such results could have significant implications for pregnant women.

Researchers at Britain's Luton University found that the Tecno AO device fixed to a VDU significantly reduced stress in users compared with the effects experienced by those using a VDU without one.

Eminent ophthalmologist Professor Mikio Miyata at Kitasato University, Japan, has shown that the Tecno AO also protected against corneal injury caused by VDU use. Analysis of the results is still continuing and will be published in a peer-reviewed journal.

While the inventor of the bioelectric shield says it works as a 'gatekeeper' to filter out incompatible energy fields, the Tecno AO antenna is thought to help the body protect itself against various frequencies by boosting brain wave frequencies to combat them. (More information and evidence is available from the Tecno AO distributor in Britain, Marketex UK, Hill Cottage, Barham, Kent CT4 6QD.)

The evidence that digital mobile phones can have serious health effects is becoming overwhelming. A researcher's case against a Welsh mobile phone distributor continues. Roger Coghill is claiming that all mobile phones should carry a label warning of possible health effects.

And in the first British legal action of its kind, a 27-year-old British woman is taking a manufacturer to court, claiming that her brain tumour was caused by radiation from her mobile phone.

Clearly, it is prudent for all of us to protect ourselves from pulsed microwave radiation, given that many of us will probably use some form of technology that generates EMR every day for the rest of our lives—which could amount to up to 40 years of exposure.

Phones are good for you

A media frenzy surrounded the "mobile phones are good for you" study and a BBC TV *Panorama* documentary presenting the research with a negative spin. The reality is that Dr Alan Preece's long-awaited research at Bristol University on the effects of mobile phone radiation on cognitive function proved to be something of a damp squib.

This was mainly due to the pathetically inadequate funding (£3000) from the Department of Health (DoH), which only allowed him to carry out two exposure tests of 25–30 minutes each on two groups of 18 subjects. Both groups were exposed to either a simulated analogue or digital mobile phone signal at 915 MHz, or no signal at all, followed by 15 different cognitive function tests.

The only significant finding, in both types of signal-exposed groups, was a 4 per cent decrease in reaction time on a choice-reaction test. Indeed, the reduced reaction time was more pronounced with the analogue phone exposure than the digital one. Different press reports interpreted this as everything from a beneficial effect to a hazard.

In fact, the result may simply have reflected the effect of the very brief exposure time in the tests. The effect may disappear or reverse with prolonged exposure in the same way that alcohol in small doses is a stimulant but, in large quantities, is a depressant.

Despite previous media misreporting, Preece did not observe any short-term memory loss (Int J Radiat Biol, 1999; 75: 447–56). However, given the small number of subjects and the limited exposure time—obvious flaws of the study—finding such a statistically robust effect on such brief exposure is worrying, especially as it could be an indication of a non-thermal effect, a possibility that both the NRPB and mobile phone industry currently deny.

Preece suggests that it might have been produced by a heating effect as the temperature in the head has been estimated to rise between 0.5 to 2 degrees C over 30 minutes when exposed to a mobile phone. But once the blood flow through the head is taken into account, a temperature rise is very small indeed—in the range of 0.01–0.1 degrees C. The NRPB generally considers a thermal effect to be one that raises the temperature by at least 1 degree C.

However, when the enhancement effect of metal—specifically, amalgam and other metal tooth-fillings, earrings and eyeglasses (especially the metal-rimmed variety)—the amount of absorption of waves could be considerably increased, causing 'hot spots' on the head that are easily above the NRPB's thermal guidelines.

This is another possibility that researchers have completely ignored to date. But, on the basis this experiment, no useful conclusion can be made—mainly because Dr Preece was not given enough funding to test the complete pulse-wave characteristics of a standard digital phone.

The real story missed by the media, and the key factor which Preece's research and that of others does not address, is the low-frequency pulsing, which a growing number of independent researchers believe is a major cause of health problems.

Pulsing effects occur below the level of heating, and are generally denied by the NRPB and the mobile industry. The non-thermal effects produced by low-frequency pulsing may be what many researchers believe are one of the principal ways that mobile phone radiation can affect brain function.

Based on previous research, notably Professor Ross Adey's findings in the US that magnetic fields can produce calcium ion influx in the brain, this low-frequency pulsing may have other effects on cognitive function. In 1994, Professor Salford in Sweden found changes in the permeability of the blood–brain barrier at levels as low as 0.016 watts/kg, which is well below the level of heating.

Recent work by Adey's long-time colleague, Dr Carl Blackman, has also shown an effect of magnetic fields on apoptosis (cell fragmentation, or programmed cell death).

It is important that any further research that the Department of Health decides to support is underwritten by enough funds to ensure some meaningful results for the 14 million Britons who currently use a mobile phone every day. Instead of a paltry £3000, it should provide something nearer to the £113,000 it was able to find for research at Porton Down's secret military research laboratory on learning deficits and changes in brain physiology in rats, the results of which will doubtless never be fully disclosed.

In the meantime, to reduce your exposure to mobile phone radiation, when you dial a number, wait until it has connected before putting the phone to your head. While searching to contact a base station, the phone is operating at a maximum strength of 2 watts.

Only once it connects does it 'power down' to about a hundredth (0.02 watts) of this level. By holding the mobile away from the head during the four to five seconds it takes to connect you will avoid your taking a four-to-five second 2-watt 'hit' to your brain every time you use it, which could spare you from an average of 10 'hits' a day.

If you are in a good reception area, the phone should automatically 'power down'. However, in an area with poor reception, the phone will stay at its near-maximum strength of 2 watts. So, when calling (or receiving) in a poor-reception area, keep the call as short as possible.

Finally, consider getting a shield or remote earpiece to cut down the radiation. Remember: you are talking about a lifetime's cumulative exposure.

Pacemaker threat

Wherever there are electromagnetic fields, there are potential problems for people with pacemakers. Mobile phones may cause problems with these lifesaving devices.

Studies have shown that some cellular phones, when placed close to implanted pacemakers, can interfere with the operation of the pacemaker (N Engl J Med, 1997; 336: 1473–9). More recent studies have shown that interference seems to occur when digital cellular phones are within three inches of the pacemaker. The interference is generally temporary and disappears when the phone is switched off or moved away from the pacemaker. However, users should be aware of the possibility of interference even when the phone is in stand-by mode.